THE Dysfluency

RESOURCE BOOK

THE Dysfluency
RESOURCE BOOK

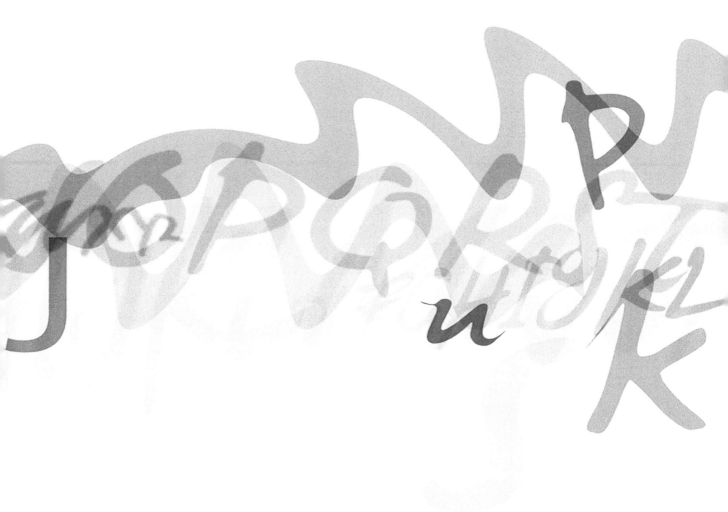

JACKIE TURNBULL & TRUDY STEWART

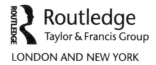

Routledge
Taylor & Francis Group
LONDON AND NEW YORK

Dedication

To all the adults we have had the pleasure of meeting in the course of our work in groups or individual therapy. You have taught us much about stammering, life and personal courage.

First published 2010 by Speechmark Publishing Ltd.

Published 2017 by Routledge
2 Park Square, Milton Park, Abingdon, Oxon OX14 4RN
711 Third Avenue, New York, NY 10017, USA

Routledge is an imprint of the Taylor & Francis Group, an informa business

British Library Cataloguing in Publication Data
Turnbull, Jackie.
The dysfluency resource book. – 2nd ed.
1. Stuttering – Treatment. 2. Stuttering –
Exercise therapy. 3. Speech therapy.
I. Title II. Stewart, Trudy.
616.8'55406-dc22

ISBN 9780863887925 (pbk)

Contents

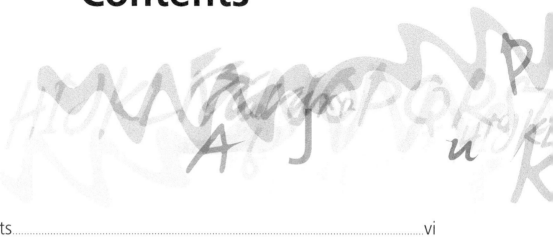

Handouts

Foreword

Stuttering (or stammering) has been a baffling problem. There have been numerous unsubstantiated theories propagated over the decades and many different approaches to its treatment arising from those theories. Few clinicians and researchers have been willing to test rigorously individual treatments and fewer still have been willing to replicate. The result has been a confusing and undesirable state of affairs. This is unfortunate because stuttering can be a serious disorder for some. By its very nature it has the potential to produce barriers to successful and 'normal' verbal communication with an attached possibility of embarrassment and frustration. Few people enjoy being too different. Furthermore, social complications can arise as a result, characterised by problems ranging from shyness and avoidance to the potentially more serious such as social isolation and depression.

Given the above, it is not surprising that the treatment of stuttering has presented a difficult challenge for many clinicians working in the area. Because of the lack of replicated research we have a deficiency of treatment protocols which provide detailed treatment guidelines. A lack of available guidelines must eventually work to lower a clinician's confidence to treat stuttering. It may also encourage the futile search for the Holy Grail of stuttering, a panacea that will resolve all our treatment problems and which will cure the problem.

So far, this Foreword has been somewhat negative. While we have ample justification to be negative, there are always reasons to be optimistic. Being an optimist at heart, I believe the tide has turned and we are now seeing excellent international efforts in resolving the difficulties associated with stuttering. *The Dysfluency Resource Book* by Jackie Turnbull and Trudy Stewart is an example of why I am positive about the future. Both authors are very experienced clinicians and have conducted research into treatment issues. They therefore have a valuable resource from which they have drawn to produce this excellent workbook for stammering. The *Resource Book* provides sufficient background material on stuttering to allow professionals to grasp the problem, and the authors provide an outstanding summary and realistic description of treatment approaches from which clinicians may choose techniques. They also provide very useful exercises and worksheets that will greatly assist clinicians working with stuttering. I believe this book is a major step forward in addressing the confusion surrounding the treatment of stuttering.

ASHLEY CRAIG
ASSOCIATE PROFESSOR
UNIVERSITY OF TECHNOLOGY, SYDNEY

Preface

The need for a 'resource' book for those managing adult clients who stammer became apparent as we listened to people asking questions. Some of these were students or clinicians less experienced than ourselves, some were beginning to specialise in dysfluency and others were just starting to practise after three or four years of training, yet their greatest concern seemed to be how to treat people who stammer and what to do. In answer to their questions, we decided to write this book.

Our aim has been to draw together information on therapy for adults, alongside practical examples of exercises, tasks and activities that can be used for individual and group programmes. We do not claim that there are any revolutionary therapeutic approaches in the book, although some of the ideas may be new to some of our readers. Rather than evaluate individual techniques and give our opinions on the various merits of each, we have tried to present a catalogue of possibilities or options from which clinicians may choose according to their clients' special requirements.

In this new edition we begin with a chapter that describes 'principles of therapy' that we believe underpin work with this client group and also gives some information on key psychological theories, which we hope clinicians will find helpful. In addition, there is a totally revised chapter on 'maintenance', subtitled 'a continuing process of change', which reflects how our thinking has changed in this area. We have also included a new chapter, 'Working in groups', in response to demands from clinicians wishing to set up groups and/or develop their practice in this area.

The ordering of the chapters relates to how we see the progression of therapy: a client will go through a process of identification, followed by desensitisation and avoidance reduction techniques before embarking on fluency-controlling strategies. Each chapter of the book follows the same format. There is a general introduction containing a brief theoretical background, then a section on how to teach the particular area, including managing possible problematic issues. This is followed by activities, many of them new to this edition, which can be used by clinicians in both individual ⓘ and group Ⓖ therapy situations. Clinicians may choose to use all the techniques, pick out particular sections, or possibly use them to familiarise themselves with specific techniques. Relevant handouts are included and these may be photocopied as required. (This is indicated by a ⓟ symbol on the pages.)

Please note that throughout, for consistency of style, the pronoun 'he' is used to refer to the client and the pronoun 'she' to refer to the clinician. In addition, again for consistency, we have used 'stammering' throughout, which can be read as 'stuttering'.

We continue to believe that there is no set 'cookbook' of ideas for working with adults who stammer. There may be a general set of principles, but each clinician will bring her own knowledge, experience and individual therapeutic style to the clinic, and this will make the application of whatever technique is chosen a unique experience for the client.

JACKIE TURNBULL
TRUDY STEWART

Acknowledgements

The idea for this book came from clinicians attending our workshops across the United Kingdom who felt a lack of confidence when working with people who stammer. They requested a manual full of 'things to do' with practical ideas, handouts and user-friendly approaches to use with their clients. We would like to acknowledge and thank them all for encouraging us to put pen to paper (or fingers to keyboard!).

In addition, we acknowledge the continuing patience and love of our families without which this book would not have been possible.

1 | Principles of therapy

We have worked with people who stammer for over 30 years. During that time we have learned a great deal from research, other clinicians, our own study and above all from clients. What any of us know about stammering is ever-changing, being challenged and redeveloped in the light of experience. This chapter represents some of our accumulated ideas and learning to date. We do not expect to feel exactly the same next month, next year or in five years' time. Indeed, we hope we do not, for it would mean that this field of study had stopped developing and that we had stopped learning.

We tell our clients that our aim is for them to end therapy being able to say what they want to say, when they want to say it, regardless of their level of fluency. How this aim is realised for each client will be unique. For some, it will involve fundamental changes in the way they construe stammering and fluency, and will entail very little, if any, change in actual speech production. For others, it will mean continuing use of techniques to control fluency and little change in their attitude to the way they speak. For most, it will be a combination of the two – a more positive approach to speaking and to the self as a speaker, reduced fear and avoidance, and the use of speech techniques in situations where increased fluency feels important. We hope that when a client ends his therapy, stammering will have become something he *does* rather than something he *is*. In other words, he will be a person first and the stammer will be just one aspect of that person.

Starting points in therapy

We work from a number of givens – attitudes, beliefs and behaviours that inform what we do.

The therapeutic relationship. There has been much discussion in recent years about the nature of the therapeutic relationship, not only in speech and language therapy but also in other caring professions (Lambert & Barley, 2001; Manning, 2000). There has been a move away from the 'medical' model in which the client comes to receive the expertise of the clinician, who has all the answers if only the client would take notice! However, we feel it is also important not to *deny* our expertise. Specialist stammering clinicians have studied their subject for many years and have learned much about its nature and about treatment approaches. Consequently, we prefer the concept of 'equal experts'. The client is the expert in his own stammering, how it affects him, how and what he wants to change and what he is prepared or able to do to allow those changes to happen. The clinician is an expert in theory and in a more generic understanding of the change process, its susceptibility to relapse and the many possible ways in which individuals experience stammering. We believe the best therapy

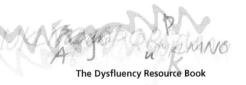

happens when the combined expertise of the client and the clinician is used. Manning uses the term 'leading from behind' to describe how this works in practice:

> We can assist him [*sic* the client] in developing new views of himself and new options concerning his fluency. With the right timing in response to changes by the client, we can help him to make better choices and to become less handicapped. We can also acknowledge that while we provide direction, insight, and information, the person who ultimately takes the lead in repairing the problem is the client.
> (2000, p226)

Work at the client's speed and from where he is in the change process. Experience and our own therapy failures have taught us how essential this is. From the very first session the clinician needs to be aware of the client's stage of change and of his perception or misconception of the therapy process. Many clients have been prevaricating over whether or not to come to therapy for weeks, months or even years and it is important that we acknowledge this huge step they have taken. For some a 'softly, softly' approach is needed, for others there is a desire to 'get the ball moving' as quickly as possible. Some may have been persuaded to come for help. Others will have fixed ideas about what therapy will entail: for example, Joanne thought group therapy would be like an Alcoholics Anonymous meeting, with each session starting with an 'I am a stammerer' confession.

It is important that we conduct a first session very carefully with all these (and more) possibilities in mind if we are to engage the client in the therapy process (if we both agree this is what is right for him at this point in time) and ensure he returns for future sessions. We will be saying more about this when we consider a 'stages of change' model later in this chapter.

Additionally, we must be aware that the speed at which someone is willing or able to change is not fixed and may not remain static throughout therapy. Someone who is very scared of change may find it so liberating when he starts to make changes that he wants to take on more challenges from quite early in therapy. Others will continue to need a more gentle and slow approach throughout therapy.

Move towards the client being his own therapist. From the outset of therapy we need to bear discharge in mind. We are working towards a time where the client does not need us and can be his own therapist. He will never achieve this status if we take all the responsibility in therapy. In order to foster this process, we encourage the client to take notes from the outset, to use what is helpful and abandon what isn't. We also want him to be honest, to tell us what he is feeling, to argue with us and tell us when he feels we are not helping or just don't understand.

Reconstruction of self as a 'fluent stammerer'. We believe it is our role as clinicians to help the client reconstrue himself as a fluent stammerer. To do this most effectively we need therefore to address not just his fluency but also his communication skills as a whole. It is of limited use if a person becomes more fluent but still feels inadequate in his ability to use verbal and non-verbal aspects of communication effectively. We are working with a person and his communication as a whole, not just the stammer in isolation.

Therapy must be informed by theory. What happens in therapy must be informed by theory (Bothe, 2004). In *Communicating Quality 3*, the Royal College of Speech and Language Therapists' guidance on best practice, service standard 23 states that 'The service has a strategic and systematic approach within each team to establish an evidence-based resource as the basis for provision of clinical care, organisation of services and service development' (2006, p116). Finn argues that an evidence-based framework should adhere to three guidelines:

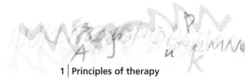

First, treatment selection is based on the best available, most recent, and clinically applicable research evidence. Second, the clinician is a self-directed learner with an appropriately critical attitude and a healthy level of scepticism about knowledge claims. Third, the person's values, concerns, and perspective are considered and evaluated throughout the selection and treatment management process.
(2003, p210)

We endeavour to adhere to these guidelines wherever possible and in the light of the evidence available to us. We have already discussed the way we consider the client's feelings about himself, his hopes for therapy and his empowerment in the process as essential to a good outcome. In the next section we discuss some of the theoretical background which underpins what we do.

How change happens

We mentioned earlier that we believe it is important to know at which stage of the change process our clients are when they present for therapy and as they proceed in their therapy journey in order to ensure therapy is appropriate for each individual. We have found the transtheoretical model of change (Prochaska & DiClemente, 1992) very helpful in this respect. The model came out of an analysis of 29 systems of psychotherapy and comprises three dimensions:

1   the levels (the 'what') of change

2   the processes (the 'how') of change

3   the stages (the 'when') of change.

The scope of this text only allows us a brief description of each of these dimensions. The model and its use in stammering therapy is described more fully in Turnbull (2000).

The levels of change

The levels relate to starting from where the client is. Prochaska & DiClemente (1992) describe five levels of change: symptom, maladaptive cognitions, interpersonal conflicts, family or systems conflicts and intrapersonal conflicts. The authors suggest that therapist and client should aim to agree the level to which the problem is attributed and at which intervention is initiated. They also propose that, wherever possible, intervention should start at the lowest level.

Some of our clients come to therapy with a very specific and limited goal in mind: for example, giving a best man's speech or saying their name on the phone. For such people, starting at the lowest level of change, that is, the symptom level, is very appropriate. Sometimes, once these clients have achieved some success with their immediate goals, they discover that there are other goals they then wish to work towards, as they see possibilities opening up which they had not previously considered. So, for example, the client who has come to therapy because he is going for job interviews where he wants more speech control (symptom level) may start to realise that he needs to look at the way he perceives his and others' beliefs about himself and his speech (maladaptive cognitions, interpersonal conflicts). His avoidance behaviours may require intervention at interpersonal, family and system levels, while his lowered self-esteem may require input at the intrapersonal level. It is important for the clinician also to be aware that levels are not independent of each other and that change at one level may well lead to change at another.

The processes of change

Prochaska & DiClemente describe ten basic change processes or types of activity 'initiated or experienced by an individual in modifying affect, behaviour, cognitions or relationships' (1986, p7). Research has shown that most systems of psychotherapy tend to utilise only two or three of these processes while self-changers typically employ eight to ten (Norcross & Prochaska, 1986). Proponents of the transtheoretical model argue that, in line with the current move to more integration and eclecticism, therapists should use a more comprehensive set of change processes and be at least as cognitively complex as their clients! Table 1.1 outlines these processes and some examples appropriate to stammering.

Table 1.1 Processes of change

Process	Description
Consciousness raising	Understanding more about stammering, for example, through overt and covert identification, observation and reading
Self-liberation	Accepting responsibility for change, making decisions
Social liberation	Seeking new alternatives in the environment, for example, by joining a self-help organisation, writing a letter to inform others
Counter-conditioning	Substituting more useful responses to difficulties, for example, by being more assertive, learning methods for anxiety control, voluntary stammering
Stimulus control	Restructuring the environment so problem behaviour is less likely, for example, by choosing not to mix with a group of people whose behaviour induces more avoidance
Self re-evaluation	Reappraising the problem, challenging unhelpful cognitions
Environmental re-evaluation	Reappraising the effect of the problem on others, for example, through asking questions of others, surveys, increased openness
Contingency management	Finding ways to reward self or get rewards from others for the changes they make
Catharsis/dramatic relief	Arousal of emotions which may previously have been repressed, for example, through role play, psychodrama or drama therapy
Helping relationships	Enlisting others to help in the change process, for example, by bringing significant others to therapy sessions and by being open about stammering

Different processes are helpful at different stages in the change process (these are discussed below). When clinicians introduce strategies that are not suitable for the stage of change the client has reached, then problems may occur. For example, self re-evaluation, dramatic relief and helping relationships are all thought to be useful processes during the stage of contemplation (Stage 2 of the model). If processes that are more suitable for the action phase are used instead, the client may feel threatened and cease attending.

The stages of change

The stages are described as 'specific constellations of attitudes, intentions and behaviours that are relevant to an individual's status in the process of change' (Prochaska & DiClemente, 1992, p5). The amount of time an individual spends in any one stage can vary considerably. Six stages are described, each one representing both a period of time and the completion of certain tasks. The stages and corresponding therapy strategies are summarised in Table 1.2.

Table 1.2 Stages of change and therapeutic interventions

Stage of change	Description	Therapist's response
Pre-contemplation	Client does not want to change	Empathy, active listening, give information, provide choices, use of paradox, give hope, remove barriers to change No treatment may be 'treatment' of choice
Contemplation	Client is 'thinking' about change but not 'doing'	Give time, weigh up pros and cons of change, explore implications of changing
Preparation	Client has made decision to change and may have made some small changes	Encourage, give autonomy, set goals
Action	Client is active in making changes	Encourage autonomy, teach skills, help client develop support networks, positive reinforcement for changes made
Maintenance	Client is keeping change going	Use of toolbox, relapse prevention plan
Termination	Client is confident of maintaining change in all situations	No therapy needed

Stage 1 Pre-contemplation

How clients present. A person at this stage is one whom therapists may describe as unmotivated, unwilling or resistant but who in reality is usually either unaware of a problem or, if aware, feels unable or unwilling to change it. He frequently denies there is a problem at all. We see few pre-contemplators and generally those we do see have been 'sent' for therapy, usually by employers or family members. Such clients frequently drop out prematurely.

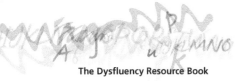

Therapy strategies. DiClemente (1991) outlines four reasons (the four Rs) why a person may choose to remain in pre-contemplation and suggests strategies that can help. *Reluctance* is often due to the person's feeling of inertia or a lack of knowledge. Empathy and appropriate feedback are useful approaches here. A client in *rebellion* is seen as having some investment in the problem behaviour and argues actively against change (perhaps it gives him a reason not to take on some difficult tasks or responsibilities). Strategies here include providing choices and possibly some careful use of paradox: for example, the therapist might say, 'It seems that you are really quite content with your speech the way it is and there is little reason for you to want to change it'. A person in a state of *resignation* does not see change as possible. The therapist's role here is to instil hope and explore perceived barriers to change. *Rationalisation* is seen when a client argues that the problem is not a problem for him. Empathy and reflective listening are seen as the most useful interventions in these cases.

When we see people in the pre-contemplation phase we are faced with some ethical dilemmas. We have to weigh up the likelihood of being able to move such clients to contemplation (the next stage of change) when we also have well-motivated clients on our waiting lists and targets to be achieved. Kuhr considers that a therapist's decision to recommend 'no treatment' can sometimes be warranted, stating that this 'requires considerable courage and the conviction that this constitutes the best course of action, given the particular circumstances' (1991, p19).

We suggest that when we are presented with a pre-contemplator and feel that attempts to move him on are likely to fail, we should consider terminating therapy but make it clear we are there to work with him if and when *he* is ready.

Stage 2 Contemplation

How clients present. A person in the contemplation phase accepts he has a problem and is thinking seriously about doing something to change it. Contemplation is characterised by ambivalence in which a client experiences both a fear of staying the same and a fear of changing. It can last for months or sometimes years. The shift from pre-contemplation tends to happen because of developmental or environmental events (for example, job prospects, relationships or the birth of a child), but unless there is also a consequent intentional change, relapse is very likely to occur.

Therapy strategies. Contemplation is not about 'doing' but about 'thinking'. It is important not to try to move the client on too quickly, but instead to give him time to weigh up the pros and cons of change. Moving the client into action too early can bring about what appears to be resistance to change and may lead to premature termination of therapy. 'Resistance' may in fact be a lack of current readiness to change, which if handled more carefully can be used to form the basis for more lasting change.

Processes found to be particularly useful at this stage include consciousness raising and self re-evaluation. Self re-evaluation techniques include encouraging a client to explore the implications of change and to weigh up the advantages and disadvantages both of staying the same and of changing. For example:

• an advantage of change: new opportunities may be opened up

• a disadvantage of change: others may expect more of the client

• an advantage of staying the same: it's safe and known

• a disadvantage of staying the same: continuing low self-esteem.

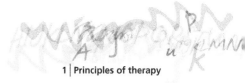

Stage 3 Preparation

How clients present. This is a short-lived stage. It combines intention and behaviour and is like a window of opportunity that will only remain open for so long; the client either has to move forward to action or back into contemplation or even pre-contemplation. The person at this stage has made a decision to change and may have initiated some tentative changes. The person who stammers may, for example, try to speak more slowly, reduce avoidance, or will tell someone about the problem. It is important that the therapist asks about any changes the client is already making in order to recognise when he is at this stage and to encourage him and so capitalise on his resolve.

Therapy strategies. Self-liberation is seen as a vital process during this stage. A client needs to believe he has the autonomy to effect change, but also to be aware that the environment can be powerful in exerting pressure on him to stay the same. Goal setting is another important strategy in the preparation stage.

Stage 4 Action

How clients present. This is where behaviour change happens. In order for change to be maintained, a client must have spent sufficient time in contemplation. However, if he stays in contemplation for too long he can lose the momentum to change. The therapist's role in the action stage is to help the client develop a sense of autonomy and take more responsibility for his own progress.

Therapy strategies. Action involves learning skills which will vary according to the level of change at which the person is: for example, if he is working at an interpersonal level he may benefit from communication skills training; if he is working at a symptom level, then specific technique work may be indicated.

It is important that clients have the support of others in their efforts to change. Some of this support can be found in group therapy, but environmental support will also be very important. Self-liberation, counter-conditioning (desensitisation, relaxation and assertiveness training), stimulus control (greater openness about stammering and enlisting friends to remind clients to act in the way they want) and contingency management (rewards for the changes that are made) are seen as necessary processes at this stage.

Stage 5 Maintenance

How clients present. A client in maintenance has made the changes he needs to make but this stage is not necessarily about keeping the status quo (see Chapter 15 'Maintenance: a continuing process of change'). It is an active stage in which change continues in order to prevent relapse. If appropriate strategies are not used in this stage relapse will occur.

Therapy strategies. Goals may change as the client realises that the changes he originally wanted to make are not those he now wants. A client can be encouraged to create his own 'toolbox', which will be essential in helping him maintain the changes he has made after therapy has ended (see Chapter 15).

Stage 6 Termination

How clients present. Termination is a more stable stage in which a client feels able to resist relapse. Four criteria are said to distinguish termination from maintenance: a new self-image,

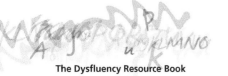

no temptation in any situation, solid self-efficacy and a healthier life style. We would argue that this stage is rarely, if ever, achieved by people who stammer and that they are likely to remain in maintenance for life.

While we have described the change cycle in a linear way, we all know that change rarely happens like that. We are sure you can think of your own examples of something you have tried to change and may have succeeded in changing: smoking, drinking, taking exercise and so on. Usually, we make lots of attempts before the change is established. We all know too of the smoker who gives up for many years and then returns to smoking at a time of stress or maybe even at a social event where the pressure to return to the old behaviour is just too much.

Typically, change occurs not sequentially but in a spiralling pattern in which there are relapses, with recycling of one or more stages. Indeed, one or more periods of relapse are seen as the norm rather than as the exception. Such relapses can be useful therapeutically as they are used to help a client be realistic and develop strategies for managing difficult times.

Theories informing psychological approaches to stammering treatment

We have said earlier that we consider ourselves to be eclectic in our approach to treatment. We draw from three particular psychological approaches, broadly based in the cognitive group of therapies, to inform our therapy approaches.

Personal construct psychology (PCP; Kelly, 1991)

Kelly proposed that a person makes sense of his world by anticipating events, using a system of personal constructs. Constructs are described as bipolar: they have two extremes that help to give them meaning. For example, someone may construe 'night' in opposition to 'day' or 'stammering' in comparison with 'fluency'. Kelly saw people as being rather like scientists who make hypotheses which they may validate or invalidate in the light of the outcome of their experiments.

Constructs are individual but can also be shared: I may have a bipolar construct of 'interesting speaker' versus 'boring speaker', which may be similar to my friend's or may be quite different. For example, the 'interesting' pole of this construct for me may mean that the person I am describing is vivacious and uses a variety of non-verbal behaviours, while the 'boring' pole may imply someone whose non-verbal repertoire is limited. My friend on the other hand may use this construct in terms of the content of the person's speech. Constructs may be 'tight' (fixed and not open to change) or loose (fluid and frequently changing). Either extreme can be seen as problematic. Constructs that are too tight can make change very difficult and frightening, whereas very loose constructs may make it hard to make any valid predictions.

PCP and stammering therapy

PCP was first used in relation to stammering by Fransella in 1972 and has been developed since by many clinicians, notably Evesham & Fransella (1985), Hayhow & Levy (1989), Fransella & Dalton (1990), Williams (1995), Stewart (1996), Stewart & Birdsall (2001). PCP is used in stammering therapy to help a client identify his constructs and, where these are unhelpful,

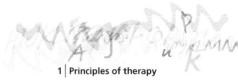

to experiment with alternatives. Some of the processes used in therapy are too involved to describe in detail here, for example, the use of repertory grids, self-characterisations and fixed-role therapy. Information about these can be found in mainstream PCP texts. We outline here a little about how PCP can be used in the process of change.

Change is seen in PCP as involving a process of loosening (thinking about and experimenting with alternative ways of construing) and then tightening (choosing from a variety of available options to explore more helpful ways of construing). Take the following example: Sam was a man of 40 who had struggled to find employment after being made redundant. He had a construct of 'needs to talk fluently' (versus 'fluency is irrelevant') with regard to prospective employers. When he stammered at interviews and did not get the job, his construing of himself at the 'needs to talk fluently' pole became even more entrenched. He was invited to consider other ways of construing his lack of success; for example, it was a difficult economic climate, he had few qualifications, he had not sufficiently prepared for the interviews, and so on. He carried out some experiments: he phoned for feedback after his next interview, he mentioned his stammer at the start of the interview, he honed his interview style through role play and advice from friends. He began to see that his original construct was in fact invalid, and that interview success was based on a range of factors, of which fluency was only one.

Cognitive behavioural therapy (CBT; Beck, 1993)

CBT was developed by Aaron Beck in the 1960s, initially as short-term therapy for depression, and has been developed since for a wide range of emotional problems. It has much in common with PCP and Beck himself talked of PCP as a forerunner of CBT. Fundamental to CBT is the view that it is our interpretation of the world that affects how we feel and behave. It is not the event that causes emotional problems per se but the meanings we give the event. So, for example, one person might think of a listener's lack of eye contact as embarrassment while another might think of it as rudeness.

CBT is a talking treatment which aims to help the person to identify and reality test unhelpful cognitions which underlie repeated negative patterns of behaviour, and to develop and test new, more adaptive cognitions that can give rise to a more positive experience of the self, others and the world (Bennett-Levy *et al*, 2004). It is structured, goal-oriented and collaborative with its emphasis on changing unhelpful thoughts and replacing them with more helpful ones. It is more concerned with how problems are maintained than on how they are caused and, wherever possible, the focus of therapy is in the present rather than the past.

CBT helps people make links between thoughts, emotions, physiological reactions and behaviours. Therapy starts with an individual formulation which the clinician and client work out together to make sense of what is happening for the client.

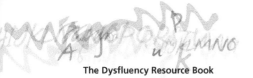

CBT and stammering therapy

A very simple formulation, taking a specific situation of asking for a bus fare, is illustrated in Figure 1.1.

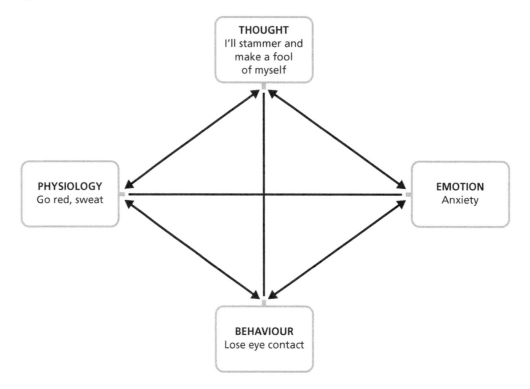

Figure 1.1 A simple formulation

In this situation the thought 'I'll stammer and make a fool of myself' leads to the emotion of anxiety, the behaviour of lost eye contact and the physiology of sweating and blushing. A vicious circle ensues: the more the person thinks he will make a fool of himself, the more anxious he gets, and the less he looks at the person, and so on.

Therapy involves helping the client first to notice unhelpful thinking and then to challenge it. The clinician uses 'Socratic questioning' in order to facilitate this process; these are questions which are open, collaborative, non-confrontational and asked with a spirit of enquiry and curiosity. Such questions do not aim to persuade the client to the therapist's point of view but rather they are used to guide discovery in the client. Below are some of the sorts of questions that can be useful in helping a client to notice and/or challenge his unhelpful thinking:

- Can you give a specific example? Who? What? Why? Where?
- How did you feel?
- What did you do?
- How is this a problem for you?
- How does 'x' go with 'y'?
- What do you mean when you say …?
- What is the evidence that … is/is not true?
- What is the worst thing that could happen if it is true?
- If it did happen, what then?

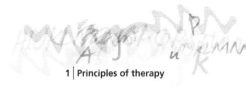
- What does this mean about how the other person thinks or feels about you?
- What does this mean about people in general?
- What would you tell a friend in a similar situation?
- What do you make of this?
- What would someone who cares about you say if they knew this?

Other questions can be used to help a client find alternative ways of thinking, for example:

- Are there any alternative explanations?
- Is the thought helpful?
- What other possibilities are just as or more valid?
- Is this thought a typical thinking error of yours?
- How can you test the thought?

CBT also uses behavioural experiments to test the validity of thoughts. Bennett-Levy *et al* (2004) divide such experiments into two types:

1 Active: once a client has identified an unhelpful cognition, he deliberately acts or thinks differently in the problem situation. This can be in a real situation or in a role play.

2 Observational: used if action is too anxiety-provoking or if more information is needed.

Experiments may be *indirect* (for example, watching a therapist voluntarily stammering in a shop) or *direct* (for example, taking part in a survey on stammering).

To summarise the main components of CBT we quote from Blenkiron:

> I think there are ten main ingredients, which are summarised below using the acronym 'CHANGE VIEW'.
>
> **C**hange: thoughts and behaviour
>
> **H**omework: between sessions
>
> **A**ct in collaboration: therapist & client
>
> **N**eed for structure: within sessions
>
> **G**oals & problems: clarify them
>
> **E**vidence based approach
>
> **V**isualise: a formulation diagram
>
> **I** can do it: self help philosophy
>
> **E**xperiments: test out beliefs
>
> **W**rite it down: to remember progress.
>
> (2007, p2)

Solution-focused brief therapy (SFBT; de Shazer, 1985, 1988)

SFBT, as its name suggests, is a forward-looking therapy based on working to a preferred future rather than on analysing problems. The term 'brief' may be confusing as in practice it really means 'as long as it takes, but not one more session than is really necessary'.

SFBT is based on a number of premises, as follows:

- Clients have resources and strengths to resolve complaints.
- Change is constant.
- The therapist's job is to identify and amplify change.
- It is usually unnecessary to know a great deal about the complaint in order to resolve it.
- It is not necessary to know the cause or function of a complaint to resolve it.
- A small change is all that is necessary: a change in one part of the system can affect change in another part of the system.
- Clients define the goal.
- Rapid change or resolution of problems is possible.
- There is no one 'right' way to view things; different views may be just as valid and may fit the facts as well.
- Focus on what is possible and changeable, rather than what is impossible and intractable.

(Adapted from O'Hanlon & Weiner-Davis, 1989, pp34–49)

In its simplest form, therapy is based on the answers to the following three key questions:

1 What does the client want?
2 What can the client do to get what he wants?
3 What needs to happen in order for the client to get what he wants?

Therapy follows a process which looks on paper to be deceptively simple and uses the following techniques:

- problem-free talk and compliments
- miracle question
- exceptions
- scaling
- what else questions
- 'getting-by' questions.

The client groups for whom SFBT is felt to be suitable include the following:

- those who have come to solve a specific problem
- those who report spontaneous recuperations
- the 'worried well' (those who have anxieties about their health which may be ill-founded)
- those with support systems
- those fed up with feeling 'stuck'.

SFBT and stammering therapy

Our training has rightly taught us a lot about analysing 'problems'. However, this approach can sometimes seem overwhelming and make the client feel that there is so much wrong that his

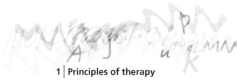

problems are insurmountable. An approach which emphasises what a client *can* do, and helps him believe that he has the resources to make changes, can be very liberating.

Looking to a preferred future helped George, a client who had had many years of therapy throughout his life, look at what he wanted and discover new ways in which he might achieve it. Using the 'miracle question' (de Shazer, 1988) showed that what he wanted was to be more confident, assertive and less fearful of starting interactions. Looking at 'exceptions' showed him that there were indeed times when he was able to be all of these things, and 'scaling' helped him look at small stages to becoming how he wanted to be more often. He started to realise that, while he might always stammer, he did not have to let his stammer determine what sort of a person he was. These processes can direct the therapist in formulating a management plan based on the client's preferred solution.

Examples of the use of all these approaches will be seen throughout the book. We advise clinicians to undertake at least some basic training in any of the approaches they are interested in using with clients.

Process and progress of therapy

The vast majority of clients who refer themselves for therapy have both overt and covert aspects to their stammering. We believe that it is essential for most clients to do at least some work on their covert issues before they are introduced to fluency-controlling techniques. Change in behaviour without a consequent change in attitude may work in the short term but is rarely maintained. In addition, when fluency-controlling techniques are taught too early in therapy they may be used by the client as a way of covering up the stammer even more.

The principal areas we address in therapy are as follows:

- identification
- desensitisation
- avoidance reduction
- fluency-controlling techniques and communication skills
- maintenance and relapse management.

Although we invariably start therapy with identification, then desensitisation and avoidance reduction, and move on later to introducing techniques, there will be times when we will additionally introduce techniques or skills training quite early in therapy. Reasons for this include the following:

- A client may have such severe overt symptoms or be so anxious about his stammering and so desperate to gain some fluency that he needs a 'carrot' to keep him engaged in the therapy process.

- There are particular overt symptoms for which more practical intervention can quickly make a difference to the person's communication, for example speaking rate, breathing patterns and the use of fillers.

- The person is at a stage of pre-contemplation or contemplation and in order to move on needs some concrete evidence that his speech can be changed through therapy.

- The nature and amount of any previous therapy and the client's attitude to it will be an important point to consider in therapy planning. If someone has had copious amounts

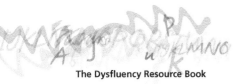

of previous therapy, then repeating stages already undertaken will be unhelpful and unnecessary.

Although it might seem that maintenance and relapse prevention work are the final phase of therapy, in fact gathering strategies to ensure skills are maintained is continuous throughout the therapy process. For example, identification is a tool which will serve the client well after therapy when he needs to carefully monitor and analyse his speech and his attitudes in order to maintain his progress. Identification will therefore also be a part of the client's maintenance plan or toolbox.

We illustrate the individual process of therapy with some brief client examples.

Client A: This young man had an extremely overt stammer. He had had a lot of previous therapy elsewhere and had learned to accept and live with his stammer. He came for therapy because he wanted some techniques to make his life easier, so that it took him less time to say what he wanted and he could keep his listener's attention. His therapy involved identification, work on breathing and fluency-controlling techniques.

Client B: This young woman's stammer was very covert. We rarely heard her stammer in the first few weeks of therapy. She needed a very gradual approach to change and to be able to make changes when she was ready, without coercion. It was important for her to spend quite some time identifying the covert aspects of her stammering, at a pace that would not feel catastrophic to her. Once she had done this she began to recognise that she needed to allow her stammer to be seen and not hidden. The process of desensitisation and avoidance reduction that followed was a long and difficult one for her which needed careful management in order to keep her engaged in the therapy process. At no point in the therapy did she work on fluency control. Her toolbox comprised ways in which she could maintain her new-found positive attitude to speaking.

Client C: This man came wanting to make sense of his stammering, not to change it. He was able to do this in individual therapy, using a PCP approach.

Client D: This man in his thirties had had some therapy elsewhere in the past. He had found it helpful and was now returning to see if there were any new techniques for him to try. He was at the stage of contemplation and used the therapy process to help him come to the decision that he did not want to move into action at present. His therapy involved mainly identification work and SFBT. The latter helped him to acknowledge that his preferred future was not dependent on increased fluency.

Client E: This student had both overt and covert aspects to his stammer. He had had no previous therapy. He worked through the stages of change in a mostly linear way, starting with identification, moving on to desensitisation and avoidance reduction. Ongoing work on identification helped him to see that some of his difficulties were not about his stammering but more to do with his verbal and non-verbal communication skills. At the technique stage he therefore worked on his posture and eye contact and also on conversational skills such as greetings and turn taking. As a student, he would return home for holiday periods and he would frequently relapse at these times. He was encouraged to use his lapses to work on relapse prevention in a very practical hands-on way and to build up a repertoire of skills which reduced his dependence on therapy to help him return to action.

Client F: This man in his forties returns to therapy every few years. He moves between action and maintenance, returning to therapy when he is ready to take on more challenges and then leaving therapy when he is ready for a further period of consolidation.

In this chapter we have described the principles that underlie our approach to stammering therapy. We go on now in the remaining chapters to describe how these approaches are realised in practice.

2 | Communication skills

Hargie points out that 'we now know that socially skilled individuals tend to be happier and more resistant to stress and psychosocial problems, and to achieve more in academic and professional contexts' (2006, p563). Stammering is not just a speech problem; it is a problem of communication. There are a number of reasons why a person who stammers may lack competence in his communication skills.

- Because of avoidance, he is less practised in communicating the things he wants to say. He may stick to situations he is sure of, in which he feels safe and about which he can make predictions.

- Because of his attitudes to speaking, a person who stammers often feels inadequate or unworthy as a communicator. He can thus appear unassertive, uninterested and/or uninteresting.

- Because of fear of stammering, a person who stammers may choose to be a 'responder' rather than an 'instigator'; he may even pretend to adhere to the same views as others because then his fluency is less likely to be disrupted.

- Fear of stammering can make a person focus on his own role in a speaking situation, thus neglecting the listener. Hence both his listening and observation skills may be impaired and the listener's feelings and thoughts are not adequately considered.

- Content is sometimes compromised because fluency is seen as the most important part of the communication.

- Over-focusing on speech and fluency can mean that non-verbal skills are ignored.

Fransella points out that:

> the stutterer knows all about playing the 'stutterer role' … he knows the variety of ways in which a person will react to his speaking, and he knows what his reactions will be to the listener's reactions. But he is inexperienced at interpreting the subtler forms of communication such as eye contact, hand gestures and general body movements, which are normal reactions to the fluent person. His focus of attention is mainly on himself, and on the degree of difficulty he is having in getting out the words he wants, and is busy interpreting the reactions of the listener, which on most occasions are reactions *to him as a stutterer*. When he speaks he construes himself as a stutterer. (1972, p58).

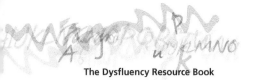
When to use

Work on communication skills may start very early in therapy. It is often less threatening for the person than working on the stammering itself. In addition, there are usually areas of a person's communication skills which will be adequate or even good and pointing these out at the start of therapy can be very affirming.

Teaching communication skills

Much of the input on communication skills will benefit from being taught in a group context, but most aspects can be considered in individual therapy and in home practice exercises. Many of the skills and deficits the person has in his communication will have been noted in the identification phase.

In this chapter we will explore three areas of communication skills: non-verbal communication (eye contact, facial expression, gesture and posture), listening and conversation skills.

Non-verbal communication

Eye contact

We will discuss later the difficulty a person may have in maintaining eye contact when he stammers (see Chapter 7 'Desensitisation'). Some people may find it difficult to look at others even when they are fluent; others may, in addition, have problems with eye contact when they are listeners. It is generally felt that the more eye contact a person uses, the more others see them as friendly. However, a person who stares at others is likely to be perceived more negatively, maybe as hostile or over-confident. Finding a happy medium can take practice. As well as helping a client develop his own eye contact, it is important to make him aware that however much he improves, some listeners will continue to look away in response, either because they find it hard to tolerate stammering or because they themselves have poor eye contact.

Facial expression

A person who stammers may show little facial expression. Perhaps this is because he is preoccupied with what he is saying or concerned with planning ahead. The aim of work in this area is to help a client to understand that by increasing his use and range of expressions, he can reinforce the meaning of what he is saying and also take his listener's focus away from fluency. It is also important that a client is aware of the links between facial expression and other non-verbal skills. For example, smiling while tapping one's foot might not convey the contentment that smiling alone would.

Gesture

Research indicates that non-verbal signals deliver five times more impact than verbal ones. If the two are not congruent, it is the non-verbal one which is most readily accepted. Gesture can be used for several purposes: instead of speech (a nod or a shrug), to enhance speech (for example, an indication of size made with the hands), an emotion (hands held up to indicate desperation, tapping one's hand to indicate boredom). For a person who stammers, gestures may also be used because use of speech alone is felt to be a problem. Someone who stammers may in addition employ gestures as a way of avoiding speech. Gestures used to enhance speech in fluent speakers may be employed not only in the same way by those who stammer, but also as a form of distraction from the dysfluency. Thus we have to ensure that any input clinicians make in this area does not merely provide more fuel for hiding or avoiding stammering.

Posture

While facial expression conveys specific information, posture conveys the intensity of the emotion. The way we stand or sit can tell others a lot about us. If, for example, we keep our head down or stand in a rigid way, others may interpret this as meaning we are unconfident or tense. We show we are well disposed to someone by assuming an open posture and perhaps by leaning forward. We can also demonstrate status by our posture; if we stand over someone we are more likely to feel in control of the situation than if we are being towered over by someone else. It is important to help a client assume postures which complement what he is aiming to communicate, rather than those which detract from or add nothing to his communication.

Activities for non-verbal communication

Group therapy is the desired forum for communication skills work. A client has the opportunity to practise skills in a situation that is closer to real life, to be given feedback from several people and to learn from others' perspectives. Most aspects can, however, be practised individually with some modification, although a client may not gain as much from one-to-one practice as he would from a group.

General *activities* for non-verbal communication skills

Note that **ⓘ** is used to indicate suitability for individual therapy and **ⓖ** for group therapy.

Discussion ⓘ ⓖ

The group discusses why is it important for a person who stammers to work on non-verbal skills. The following points should emerge, but if not the clinician should raise them.

- Feeling more competent as a communicator will increase confidence in speaking.

- Acting *as if* one is confident can bring about responses in others, which in turn increase *actual* confidence.

- Concentrating on other skills takes the emphasis off the stammer, for both the speaker and the listener.

- If the person communicates well he is more likely to hold the listener's interest.

- The person is likely to enjoy speaking more if he feels he performs well.

It may be useful to give clients a handout on non-verbal behaviour (see Handout 1).

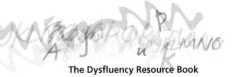

Silent communication ⚙

This activity can help to demonstrate how much information can be delivered without the need for words. In pairs or in a group, participants take it in turns to communicate something to their partner or the rest of the group. It is the ideas and not any specific words that must be guessed. The observers have to guess what the message is as quickly as they can. The person whose mime has been guessed most quickly is the winner. Examples of subjects to communicate might be:

- I am sad because my dog has died
- I am feeling ill
- My mother has gone on holiday
- The weather is fantastic
- House prices are rising
- My friend has won the lottery
- I am late for the cinema.

Home-based activity 1

The client watches people he comes across in his everyday life, as well as people in the media, and returns to therapy with lists of good and bad communication skills.

Home-based activity 2

The client evaluates himself as a communicator, listing those things he feels he is good and not so good at. He can supplement his own observations by asking the views of friends and other group members if appropriate and by analysing his own performance on video.

Activities for specific non-verbal communication skills

Once a client has a good understanding of desired skills, he can look at those he feels are particularly relevant for him to practise. It should be pointed out to a client that many people who do not stammer have poor communication skills for a variety of reasons. They may, for example, be lacking in confidence, uncertain of what they are saying, inexperienced in talking in many situations or come from a background where communication is not considered an important skill.

It is important to be sensitive to the differences in non-verbal behaviours between cultures. Some cultures, for example, see it as unacceptable to look someone in the face, while in others the 'personal space' required by individuals is considerably less than might be acceptable, for example, in the UK.

Activities for eye contact

Discussion ⓘ ⚙

What constitutes good eye contact? Using information gleaned from observation exercises in the previous section, ideas to consider could include the following:

- There is a difference between appropriate eye contact and staring.

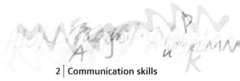

- The amount of eye contact can have different implications: for example, more eye contact can represent both intimacy and supremacy, depending on the context.

- An averted gaze can indicate fear, untrustworthiness, boredom, lack of confidence, or that the person is thinking.

- The most helpful pattern is of frequent eye contact interspersed with looking away. The ratio of the glances will vary considerably according to the situation: for example, on a train the glances are likely to be infrequent and momentary, with a close friend the eye contact will be more frequent and maintained for longer.

Role play ⬤ ⚙

With the clinician or with other group members, a client or group of clients is given situations to role play. Other group members and/or the clinician observe and give feedback on the appropriateness of the amount of eye contact given for the specific situation. If it is a group situation, comments can also be made about the distribution of the eye contact among the listeners. Situations might include:

- talking to a close friend or family member

- attracting someone's attention

- asking for a ticket

- making a complaint

- at a bar in a nightclub

- an interview

- giving a presentation

- introducing two people

- asking for directions

- at a supermarket checkout.

Discussion ⬤ ⚙

Handout 2 'Increasing eye contact when stammering' is used as a basis for discussion.

Monologue ⬤ ⚙

The client is asked to talk about his job, a holiday or a hobby (something fairly unemotive). The aim is for him to initiate eye contact just before he begins to speak. This helps him to establish his speaking turn and then to maintain eye contact once speaking begins.

Speaking circles ⚙

This activity, described fully in Chapter 7 'Desensitisation', is a powerful exercise which aims to help people feel at ease when using eye contact in a group.

Home-based activity

This exercise is for a client who has difficulty in maintaining eye contact as a listener. He is asked to notice specific things about another person's face. To make this activity more interesting you could use the 'People's bingo' sheet we have included as Handout 3, or make one up specific to your client's needs.

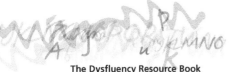
Activities for facial expression

Expressing emotions facially ⓘ ⓖ

Sentences are written on cards placed face down in a pile. A client chooses an emotion to express and reads the sentence using an appropriate facial expression. Listeners have to guess the emotion. Some sample sentences are given on Handout 4 'Sentences for facial expression exercise'.

Home-based activity 1

The client is asked to observe people around him and in the media and return to therapy with examples of how facial expression impacts on the message and affects the listener. The resulting discussion should focus on (1) the match (or mismatch) of expression between speaker and listener, (2) the intensity of expression (too much or too little), (3) the effect of limited expression, and (4) the way in which facial expression impacts on the conversation (that is, how it carries emotion rather than content). The feedback sheet (Handout 5) can be used to record the client's findings.

Home-based activity 2

The client is asked to watch the television or a DVD with the sound turned down and try to ascertain the content area (*what* is being said) and the emotion behind the words (for example, abstract, emotional, intimate, distant, academic). If a DVD is used, it can be replayed to see how successful the guesses were. In most cases it will transpire that the words carry the actual message but the expression carries much of the emotion.

Activities for gesture

Discussion ⓘ ⓖ

Handout 6 'Gesture' can be used for information and discussion.

Range of gestures ⓘ ⓖ

Each group member in turn performs a commonly used gesture (such as shoulder shrugging, hand rubbing). Another client or the clinician identifies the implied meaning of the gesture. The activity ends when no more meanings can be thought of. The purpose of the activity is to demonstrate the enormous range of gestures in common usage. Alternatively, and in individual therapy, gestures can be written on cards for a client to act out. Ideas for cards are given on Handout 7.

Identifying gestures ⓖ

In front of the group, each member has to demonstrate something he did the day before, by using gesture alone. The other group members have to guess the activity. More subtle activities can be put on cards for a participant to act out (refer to Handout 8). This exercise demonstrates just how much information can be gleaned without the use of speech.

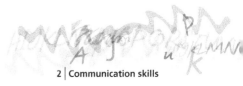

Activities for posture[1]

Discussion 🛈 🝢
Handout 9 'Good posture' is used to inform and as a basis for discussion.

Using posture 🝢
Group members are given cards on which specific postures are described (see Handout 10 'Posture exercise'). In pairs, they carry out a conversation using the given posture and report back to the group the effect, if any, this had on both participants.

Posture questionnaire 🝢
Handout 11 'Posture questionnaire' is used by group members working in pairs. Each member reports back on his partner's posture. Areas to work on can then be targeted for home practice.

Home-based activity 1
Handout 12 'Posture: home practice' is given out and then used as a basis for follow-up discussion on the effect of posture on the listener, the speaker and on speech.

Home-based activity 2
A client observes people speaking to one another at a distance, where the words cannot be heard, and is directed to watch their posture. A television programme or DVD can also be used for this exercise. From others' posture a client aims to ascertain the following:

- how each person in the conversation is feeling
- if one person is in control
- whether all participants are being honest
- if the atmosphere is generally friendly or unfriendly
- the status of each participant in the group.

Home-based activity 3
A client experiments with different postures (using Handout 10 'Posture exercise' if appropriate) and observes what effect the postures have on the listener and on his communication. He may, for example, stay standing while having a conversation with a seated boss, sit forward to show interest in what someone is saying, slouch in a chair with feet on a coffee table. The results of these experiments can be discussed in therapy sessions.

Listening skills

Often people who stammer tell us they are good listeners. They sometimes base this on the fact that they are generally less active in conversations than more fluent speakers. We would question whether silence and listening are synonymous and suggest that often when people who stammer are quiet, it is because there is too much inner activity going on for them to be able to focus sufficiently on the other person. They may instead be planning their next word, working out if they do actually have to speak, and if so, whether they can change any of their words. To be a good listener it is not enough to be quiet; the person must actively listen and demonstrate by their behaviour that they are doing so.

---

[1] Our thanks are due to Lisa Gill and Justine Ben-Yosef, who at the time of writing were 3rd year speech and language therapy students on placement with us. They carried out a session on posture for our group and are responsible for the posture handouts in full or in part.

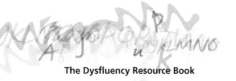

Activities

Brainstorm 🔅

Brainstorm 'features of a good listener'. Alternatively, this exercise could be introduced as a question: 'If you were to watch a video of a good listener with the sound turned off, what would you see?'

Trios exercise 🔅

In threes (speaker, listener, observer), with each participant performing each role in turn, the speaker tells of a recent event that has concerned him. The listener has to practise good listening skills. The observer checks on the 'Observer checklist' (Handout 13) those skills that have been used and notes any that have been omitted. Alternatively, clients first identify specific skills they wish to have monitored.

Discussion 🔅

The group has a discussion on a given subject, preferably one that is emotive and likely to encourage a lot of participation. The rule is that no one can make his point without first summarising what the person before him has said. At the end of the discussion, reference can be made to statistics that show that we only remember about a quarter of what is said to us.

Story reading 🔅

Four or five volunteers are requested for this activity. They are taken out of the room and one is given a short story to read and remember (see Handout 14 'Story for listening exercise'). This person and one of the other volunteers are brought back into the room and the one who read the story is instructed to retell it to the other. The rest of the group use Handout 15 'Checklist for listening exercise' to help them spot which points are remembered and which are forgotten in the telling of the tale. The next volunteer is then brought in and the person who has been told the story has to repeat the version he has been told (which is usually rather different from the original!). This process is repeated by each of the volunteers in turn, who tell the story as they have just heard it. The last person tells the story to the whole group. Once the story has been told by the last volunteer, feedback is given to each of them as to the kind of things they remembered and the things that were forgotten. In our experience, the following things are noticed in most groups:

- The beginning of the story seems to be more easily remembered than the end.
- Names, eg 'Dagenham', 'Ford', are often recalled.
- Trivial information may or may not be recalled.
- If the actual sense is lost, people try to make their own sense of it and will reinvent the story, adding and leaving out bits of the original in order to do so.
- People vary a great deal in their ability to recall.
- A written story is more easily remembered than a spoken one.

Home-based activity

A client uses the 'Listening skills observation exercise' (Handout 16) to find examples of good and bad listening skills in his everyday life.

Activities for monitoring the listener

Using 'soaps' ⓘ 🅖

In this activity, a pre-recorded excerpt from a soap such as *EastEnders, Hollyoaks or Coronation Street* is used. A client looks at the recording with the volume turned off and is then asked, on the basis of the body language, to interpret (1) what the characters may be saying, (2) what they are wanting to say but not actually saying, and (3) what they are feeling. A client should support his opinions with specific behavioural examples such as, 'He is feeling angry. He is standing close to her and staring at her hard. He is also using threatening gestures, such as finger pointing. I think he is saying something like "I am warning you"'.

Home-based activity

The client chooses one conversation per day when talking to someone with whom he feels comfortable. He listens and looks for one of the following:

- What does the person say to indicate he has not understood?

- What does he say to encourage the client to continue to speak?

- What signs are there that the other person may have lost the thread of what the client is saying?

- What clues are there that the other person is finding what the client is saying of particular interest?

Conversation skills

An adult who stammers will have spent many years adapting his conversation in order to try to hide or avoid stammering. As a result, conversations may be cut short, social niceties may be omitted, or, because of avoidance levels, a person may lack the practice to develop skills in some basic areas. There are times when, in addition to looking at non-verbal communication, we also need to help a client learn to converse better. We are certainly not suggesting that people who stammer are the only ones who can benefit from such training, nor that all who stammer need it. There are many people in the general population who lack skills in certain areas. Here we merely present a few ideas as to what might be covered if input in this area is felt to be necessary.

Conversation skills training is clearly most effective as part of a group therapy programme and can be used at any stage in the therapy process. We find the topic is best introduced as a 'theme' which is covered in one or two sessions and then followed up by a client devising his own targets, based on what he has learned from the sessions about his own conversation skills. For example, if he finds starting off a conversation particularly difficult, then this will be the area he will work on.

These skills can also be taught once a client has learned techniques for controlling his stammering, but may still need practice in order to integrate them into conversation. Having to think about what to say as well as using a technique can be hard, and these exercises provide useful practice in a safe environment.

This is a huge subject and we are only able to cover some basic topics which clinicians can then use to select and develop ideas and activities. It is useful to break conversation into specific component parts. We have found the following useful areas to consider: greeting, starting and keeping a conversation going (initiating/changing/continuing topics) and parting.

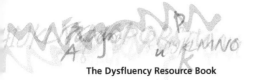
Teaching conversation skills

Greetings and introductions

For someone who stammers, greetings and introductions can be fraught with anxiety. Specific words are generally required ('Hello', 'Good morning'), and perhaps a name has to be said which cannot be avoided or changed. Often the spoken part is felt to be so difficult for the person who stammers that he does not even consider the impact of non-verbal aspects, such as facial expression, eye contact, proximity and so on.

Activities

Discussion ⚙

Discuss non-verbal aspects of greetings. A client explores how a person shows someone his intentions as he approaches others. This exercise can be extended by having two lists of cards, one with situations written on and the other with methods. A client takes one card from each pile and tries to act the two out together. Some will fit together and be appropriate, others will not, and this can be discussed. Here are some ideas for cards:

Intentions

friendly

in a hurry

wanting a long chat

wanting a brief chat

unfriendly towards the person

embarrassed at seeing them (perhaps you should have contacted them before).

Methods

smiling

frowning

looking at your watch

looking down

using good eye contact

talking while moving

stopping

showing little facial expression

starting a topic of conversation.

Opening statements ⚙

In a circle, a ball is thrown to a group member, who makes some sort of greeting or introductory statement such as 'Hello, isn't it a lovely day?', 'Hi, I've not seen you in ages', 'How are you doing?', 'I'm Jackie', 'I'm Trudy. Haven't we met somewhere before?' The person who catches the ball has to throw it to another group member, who gives a different opening response. The exercise continues until each group member has had several turns or messages start to be repeated. In this way, clients have the opportunity to 'play about' with different remarks and see what they feel comfortable with. In our experience, clients often seem to feel almost that they are 'compelled' to use a very limited set of words and that they are 'cheating' if they use any other. This exercise can show the range of acceptable opening gambits that are actually available. The implications of avoidance behaviours need to be discussed too; there can be little difference sometimes between 'experimentation' and avoidance.

Role play ⚙

Role play different sorts of greetings and appropriate non-verbal and verbal behaviours. Situations could include the following:

- being introduced to someone new at work: a boss, a colleague or a visitor

- meeting someone at a social event whom you have met before and would like to get to know better

- meeting an old friend and wanting to re-establish a relationship

- running into someone you know only slightly

- meeting someone you do not like but with whom you feel the need to be civil but not over-friendly

- going into a local shop

- meeting a new neighbour for the first time.

Introductions in a social or public setting ⚙

In this type of setting, introductions are usually made in one of two ways: a request for information, such as 'Do you have the time?' or 'Can you show me how to work this machine?', or through the use of conventional asides such as 'Isn't it a lovely day?' or 'Wasn't it a great game?' These can be role played, with appropriate responses to indicate whether the other person wants to continue, such as a furthering of the topic or a return to a newspaper after a brief response.

Getting the conversation going

Breaking the ice with the use of 'non-task' topics is often a good way of starting a conversation. Subjects such as the weather, uncontroversial aspects of the latest news and comments about the specific situation people are in are the most common subjects. It may be useful to point out that many people are trained to use such strategies for a variety of reasons, for example, a doctor or dentist (to put the patient at ease) or a salesman (to engage the person before moving in with the real intent).

Activities

Role play activities for ice breaking

Public setting ℹ ⚙

- A doctors' surgery: people arrive sporadically for their appointments, first giving their name and appointment time to the receptionist. They sit down in the waiting room. Ice-breaking activities are initiated. The receptionist announces that the doctor has been delayed.

- A bus stop: the bus is already 10 minutes late and it is a cold day. Each participant is given a card with an ice-breaking remark he has to introduce into the conversation: for example, 'These buses are never on time', 'The shops will be closed by the time I get there', 'They say it's going to rain later on'.

Private social setting 🛈 🎛

- A wedding reception: the photos are being taken. As above, participants have cards with remarks they must use: for example, 'Doesn't the bride look beautiful?', 'Is it a buffet or a sit down meal?', 'I do hope it doesn't come on to rain'.

These activities obviously work most effectively in a group. They can, however, be adapted for use in individual therapy. Therapist and client can together compile a list of ice breakers and then use the situations above to role play short snippets of conversation, using the ideas they have elicited. We have also press-ganged secretaries, receptionists and other therapists into taking part in these role plays!

Keeping the conversation going

Conversations can, of course, end at any point. Some get no further than the greeting: for example, 'Hello, how are you?', 'Fine thanks, yourself?', 'Fine'. Others stop at the ice-breaking stage. As conversations proceed, 'meshing' skills are used. These bring speaker and listener skills together. It can help to think of three areas for conversations: content, timing and turn taking. Understanding how these areas work together in conversations can help people who lack confidence in communication to have a structure on which to base their conversations, and to identify and work on any problem areas.

Content

Content refers to 'what' is said and to how ideas expressed continue or change.

Timing

The normal pattern for timing is that one person speaks and when they stop the other person starts to talk without undue silence or interruption. Stammering can affect timing adversely. One scenario is that the person who stammers leaves an over-long gap before he takes his conversational turn (as discussed below). Another scenario is that the listener interrupts him when he is stammering, for a variety of reasons. He may think that the person has finished talking, be embarrassed at the silence, or try to supply a word that the person who stammers is getting stuck on.

Turn taking

When someone stammers, turn taking can be especially problematic, because of difficulties in initiating and sometimes in terminating speech. Often there is a sense of urgency in what the person who stammers says; a feeling that once started, he has to finish at all cost. Developing strategies to make turn taking easier can give the person more of a sense of control.

Activities

Activity for content

Discussion ⓘ ⚙

Handout 17 'Keeping the conversation going' is given as a basis for discussion. In group therapy, clients can break into pairs to practise these ideas. A client can be given starting sentences, examples of which are given below.

- I really hate Christmas shopping.
- I am finding it very difficult with my son. He is being really naughty.
- I am so looking forward to some time off.
- There is a yet another supermarket opening near us.
- I went to a great new restaurant the other day.
- I really like watching Formula One. It's so exciting.

Alternatively, a client is given a theme such as 'leisure' and experiments with each of the three styles discussed in the handout, looking at the relative value of each: (1) disclosing similar information, thoughts and ideas about a similar topic, (2) talking about a similar topic but disclosing different information and/or feelings, and (3) maintaining the same feelings but changing the topic.

Activities for timing

Discussion ⓘ ⚙

Discuss turn taking and reasons why 'correct' patterns of turn taking do not always occur. The following are just a few possibilities.

- One person is not listening to the other.
- The listener does not notice or pay attention to 'hand-over cues', such as reduced eye contact, lowered pitch, forward body posture.
- The listener does not know what to say.
- The listener is too eager to get his point across.

Mistiming ⓘ ⚙

One person speaks and the other gets the timing wrong: he either interrupts or leaves it too long before responding. The effect on the listener is discussed.

Activities for turn taking

Video ⚙

Pairs of clients have a conversation which is videoed. The videos are played back and group members observe the turn-taking skills used well and less well.

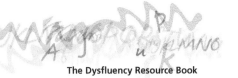

Discussion ⓘ ⚙

Discuss the specific difficulties of silence due to stammering. Ideas are generated as to how to deal with these (refer to the section on dealing with silence in Chapter 7 'Desensitisation').

Social routines

Social routines are used in order to confirm and support relationships. They include giving and receiving praise, compliments, support, encouragement, help, apologies, congratulations and sympathy.

Activities for social routines

Discussion ⓘ ⚙

Discuss which social routines a client finds easier and which more difficult to express. Consider the relevance of the stammer to this. In a group setting, each can be role played and feedback given.

Specific social routines

Giving compliments ⚙

In a circle, group members take it in turns to pay a compliment to the person on their right. That person has to respond appropriately. For example, person A says, 'That's a lovely outfit you are wearing', to which person B replies, 'Thank you. I like it too' (and not, 'What, this? It's an old thing I've had for years').

Offering support and encouragement ⓘ ⚙

Group members (or the therapist in individual therapy) are given cards with good and bad statements written on. Other members (or the client in individual therapy) have to make an appropriate response. Examples of openers could be:

- I've won the lottery.
- My grandfather has just died.
- I've got a new kitten.
- My wife is pregnant.
- My car has been vandalised.
- My son has been made redundant.
- I have a stammer.

Offering help and receiving offers of help: discussion ⚙

Ideas are pooled on how to offer help and how to accept or refuse politely. Difficulties clients have in this area, especially relating directly to stammering (such as finding specific words or people difficult to talk to), are discussed. Clients and therapist take turns to think of alternative ways of behaving. These can also be role played if only two participants are required.

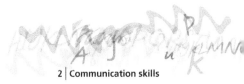

Role play

Situations can be role played in which one person offers help to another and the other refuses or accepts. Real-life experiences which group members have encountered can be used as an alternative or addition. These situations can be played in the same way as they happened, and then, after discussion, as the person would now aim to carry them out. Ideas for situations are:

- Someone is going on holiday. Their neighbour offers to look after the dog, or check the newspapers and milk are not delivered, or go in and draw the curtains.

- A person's car breaks down. Someone offers to drive them to their destination in their own car, or call the breakdown services, or lend them their car.

- One person asks another for a loan of £20.

Offering congratulations: discussion

Discuss the non-verbal and verbal responses which may be used and the appropriateness of each in different situations and with different people: for example, 'Well done', 'Good on you', 'Congratulations', 'I knew you'd do it', a pat on the back, handshake, smile. In a group setting, two subgroups could each identify such behaviours under the headings 'non-verbal responses' and 'verbal responses'. These behaviours are then put on cards and group members in turn pick up a card from each pile and act out a situation they have encountered where congratulations were in order. The clinician and/or other group members comment on the appropriateness of the verbal and non-verbal responses for the person to whom they are given.

Role play

Look at ways in which someone might handle a situation where congratulations are in order but the person giving the congratulations has reservations about the situation. Possible situations to role play might be:

- One person tells a good friend he has become engaged. The other person may or may not like the fiancée.

- It is your parents' wedding anniversary. They have/haven't been getting on too well recently.

- Your best friend has a promotion. He will have to move away.

- A member of a sports group to which you belong tells you he has been asked to play in a higher league.

Closure

Merely stopping talking is not an adequate way of ending a conversation. There needs to be some form of closure which takes place and is recognised by both parties. The type of closure used will depend upon a wide range of factors, such as whether the relationship is to continue and, if so, on what basis, whether both people are in agreement as to the timing of the parting, the background and expectation of both parties, and so on.

There are four ways a conversation can be closed:

1 factual – as in a summary or a conclusion

2 motivational – a suggestion of an idea to ponder

3 social – such as leaving the conversation showing it has been of use ('I've enjoyed talking to you')

4 perceptual – for example, a verbal closure ('Goodbye') or a non-verbal closure (taking a step back).

Understanding this routine may help a person who stammers to place less emphasis on the final words of parting, which can be a particular concern if those words are feared. Some people who stammer find it hard to end conversations for this reason and may prolong them unduly.

Activities for closure

Routines ⓘ ⚙

In pairs, people work out possible routines. Clinicians can first demonstrate with an example, such as the following:

Person A: Well, I think I've got a good idea now about the sort of computer I should be looking for.

Person B: It might be a good idea to buy a magazine to see what meets those specifications at your price.

Person A: Thanks a lot for your help.

Person B: It's a pleasure. I look forward to seeing you again. Cheerio for now.

Person A: Bye!

Clients should use situations from their own experience for this exercise.

Use of recorded extracts ⓘ ⚙

The clinician videos 'partings' from films, media interviews and so on. Alternatively, two clinicians can role play partings in front of the group. A client is instructed to be aware of the non-verbal as well as the verbal aspects of the final parting. A client observes and makes a list of the non-verbal ways people show they are parting. The list is likely to include the following:

• a parting position, such as standing up if seated, moving towards a door or moving back

• a handshake

• a touch on shoulder

• a kiss

• a smile

• a wave.

It should be pointed out that sometimes there is no need for a specific 'goodbye' word.

Brainstorm ⓘ ⚙

Brainstorm all the possible words or phrases which can be used in parting, such as 'goodbye', 'cheerio', 'cheers', 'adieu', 'auf wiedersehen', 'au revoir', 'ciao', 'bye', 'goodnight', 'ta-ta' and so on. The suitability of each for different situations can be discussed.

Home-based activity

A client 'tries out' parting words he does not usually try and reports back on how they were received and how he felt saying them.

Non-verbal behaviour

It is estimated that the verbal (what we actually say) aspects of speech carry one-third of social meaning, while the non-verbal aspects carry two-thirds. Working on this aspect of communication can therefore pay dividends.

What is non-verbal behaviour?

It includes vocal behaviour (tone of voice, rate of speech, volume, intonation) and also facial expression, gesture, eye contact and posture.

What is it used for?

1   It can be used to give messages without speaking: for example, a smile when someone sits down next to you on the bus tells them that what they have done is acceptable.

2   It is also used to say more than the words themselves. It conveys the emotion attached to the words or reinforces the message: for example, we may say something is big but a gesture with our hands can show just how big.

3   Some gestures are used to contradict the verbal message: for example, a school child may say 'Yes Sir' when asked if he is sorry for a misdemeanour, but the confident way in which he stands implies he is far from sorry!

4   Non-verbal communication can be used by a person to indicate that he has finished talking and is giving his 'turn' to someone else, for example, by lowering his volume, changing pitch or looking at the person.

5   It may be used to give feedback, for example, showing concern or joy through facial expression, gesture or touch.

Routledge
Taylor & Francis Group

Increasing eye contact when stammering

A person who stammers often finds it difficult to look at the person he is speaking to. This may be caused by embarrassment or fear of seeing an adverse reaction. However, very often poor eye contact only serves to increase the listener's own embarrassment and to make a negative reaction more likely.

Increasing eye contact when you are stammering is not easy. You are likely to have been reacting in this way for several years and it has probably become a well-established habit. The following steps can help:

1   Work first on your eye contact as a listener. Observe people as they are talking to you. You may find it easier to do this if you set yourself a task, such as looking for the colour of their eyes, the shape of their nose, the size of their ears and so on.

2   Look at yourself in a mirror at home. You might want to start by 'pretending' to stammer. Throw yourself into a really big block or repetition and keep looking at yourself. Do this until you can do it without feeling anxious. For your next step you might have a conversation with someone close to you (having told them first what you are planning to do) and then look in the mirror as you talk to them, making sure you keep eye contact with yourself when you stammer. Again, keep doing this until your anxiety subsides.

3   Now have the conversation but look directly at the person. Ask them to tell you if you look away during a stammer.

4   Using the mirror again, make a telephone call and maintain eye contact in the mirror.

5   Try to use good eye contact with other people. Start with those you find it easiest to talk to. You may find it helpful to tell them what you are trying to do and to ask them to remind you if you start to look away when you stammer. Work up gradually, trying it out with increasingly 'difficult' listeners. If they avoid eye contact with you, try not to let it deter you from keeping eye contact with them.

6   Try and increase the number of people you use your good eye contact with. Set yourself targets and increase them gradually. Slowly but surely you will learn to replace your bad habit with a good one. Don't expect to change the habits of a lifetime overnight, but do expect to change them in time!

Routledge

People's bingo: eye contact exercise

When you speak to someone during the week ahead, observe one of the following and record your observations on the sheet as soon as possible after the conversation.

The colour of their eyes	Are they wearing make-up?	The shape of their head	The number of times they smile
The bushiness of their eyebrows	The size of their ears	Are they wearing earrings?	Do they wear glasses?
Is their eye contact appropriate?	Their hairstyle	The colour of their hair	The length of their eyelashes
The length of their hair	How prominent are their cheekbones?	Their most obvious facial feature	The size of their nose

Routledge
Taylor & Francis Group

Sentences for facial expression exercise

You make me so angry when you do that

That's absolutely amazing!

That is a terrible thing to have happened

You must be thrilled

Just get out and don't come back

I've had a terrible shock

I've passed all my exams with distinction

I'm feeling really faint

I've booked a trip to Florida

Whatever did you do that for?

My friend is expecting triplets

Leeds United won the Cup Final

I can't find my wallet anywhere

Can't you do anything right?

Where on earth have you put that book?

I wish you weren't going

It's ages since I've seen you

I can't stand her

I told you so

Routledge

Feedback sheet

Person you observed, eg friend, relative, person being interviewed on TV	Did the speaker seem genuine?	How well did the speaker's facial expression match what they were saying?	Did the speaker use too much/too little/ the right amount of facial expression?	How well did the listener's expression match the speaker's facial expression?

Gesture

Gesture is thought to be used for four main reasons:

1   Instead of speech – these sorts of gestures (for example, nods, shrugs of the shoulders, a 'thumbs up' signal or a wave of the hand) are generally universally understood within a culture. They may be used as a form of shorthand or in situations where speech is more difficult (for example, a noisy or quiet environment, or when someone is some distance away).

2   To make speech more descriptive – for example, we may say something is small but if we indicate the size with our fingers it makes it more real and in some cases more dramatic.

3   To show our feelings about something – for example, we may take a step back in disgust or put our arms around someone to show we care.

4   Some gestures, often used without our conscious awareness, are those which express our feelings, often when we are finding it difficult to manage them. Twisting our hair may, for example, be an indication of anxiety, while tapping our fingers may illustrate boredom.

All these gestures are widely used by all speakers, fluent or not. For a person who stammers, however, sometimes they are over- or under-used.

Over-use of gesture may be because a person:

• is trying to distract the listener from their speaking

• feels their speaking is not adequate to express what they want to say

• wants to avoid speaking as much as possible.

Under-use of gesture may be because a person:

• the person is anxious about communication as a whole

• has considerable body tension

• prefers not to draw attention to himself in any way.

When working on gesture, it is important to be aware of the following:

1   It is important not to use either too much gesture, which can be distracting for the listener, or too little, which can make you appear tense or less interesting.

2   The same gestures may have different meanings in different settings and in different cultures.

3   Gesture should not be forced, but should feel and look natural.

4   Gestures should match your feelings; if they do not, other people may become suspicious about what you are saying.

Routledge
Taylor & Francis Group

Gesture cards

Rub your hands together

Shrug your shoulders

Thumbs up

Thumbs down

Pretend to throw salt over your shoulder

Wring your hands together

Throw your head back in the air

Scratch your head

Suck/bite your fingers

Put your index finger on your chin

Hold a clenched fist in the air

Place both hands on your hips

Point your finger at someone

Stick out your tongue

Screw up your face

Put your hand over your eyes

Hold your hand out to be shaken

Nod your head

Shake your head

Clap your hands

Raise your eyebrows

Tap your fingers repeatedly on your knee or on the table

Bite your bottom lip

Suck in your cheeks

Routledge
Taylor & Francis Group
ROUTLEDGE

Activities to act out using gesture alone

Talking to an elderly, deaf person

Talking to a young child

Teaching a child to ride a bike

Listening to someone in a noisy pub

Being examined by a doctor

Examining a rash on your arm

Buying a watch

Buying ingredients for a cake

Buying a hat

Watching a violent TV programme

Watching a sentimental film

Having a candlelit dinner for two

Queuing for a bus

Arguing at a counter about a mistake the bank has made

Sitting through a boring concert

Waiting for an important phone call

Visiting someone with a newborn baby

Waiting to have a painful tooth extracted

Asking a favour

Apologising for a serious mistake

Good posture

There are many benefits to good posture:

1   It is a basis for good breathing, which is essential for speech production

2   It helps you to move in an efficient manner

3   It ensures your internal organs are not restricted and helps with circulation

4   It keeps your bones and joints in the best position for your muscles to work well

5   It adds strength or increased meaning to what you are saying

6   It helps you look confident

7   It helps you feel more in control

Good standing posture

• Keep your body aligned: stand as if you have a string fixed to the top of your head which is keeping you erect

• Try to feel your spine lengthen and do not slump or round your shoulders

• Keep your head central in your body with your chin up but not tense

Good sitting posture

• Where possible use a chair that is at a good height to support your back and allow your feet to rest flat on the floor

• Do not slouch

• Keep your shoulders relaxed and dropped down slightly (not hunched)

At work

• Try not to hold the phone between your head and your shoulder as this can cause tension

• If you use the phone a lot it would be beneficial to use a special headset

• Make sure any computer screens and chairs you use are at the correct height to avoid strain

Routledge
Taylor & Francis Group

Posture exercise

Stand up straight

Sit slouched

Sit rigidly

Lean forward

Sit with your feet on another chair

Clasp your hands behind your head

Face away from the listener

Fold your arms and legs tightly

Stand and keep moving from one foot to the other

Sit with your legs on another chair

Rock back and forth on your chair

Sit the wrong way round on the chair

Stand with your hands on your hips

Routledge

Posture questionnaire

In pairs, ask each other questions about *your own* posture, generate ideas and be prepared to feed back to the group about your partner.

1 What aspects of my posture do you think are good?

2 What aspects of my posture do you think I need to work on?

3 Do you think that my posture affects my speech and/or communication in any way?

4 What message does my posture give out to other people?

5 Can you give me one practical tip to help me improve my posture?

Routledge
Taylor & Francis Group

Posture: home practice

As a starting point to working on your posture, try out each of these postures when you are in conversation.

Use them at varied times in your regular day-to-day activities (eg at work, at home, in the pub) and with a varied range of people (eg friends, family, colleagues, strangers). Try and do each one for about five minutes and note down the following:

(i) The effect it has on your **speech** and **communication** as a whole (include **how others react to you**).

(ii) At least one adjective to **describe a person displaying that posture** (eg lazy, confident, rude).

Be prepared to discuss with your clinician and/or other group members!

1 Sitting slumped forward in a chair, shoulders hunched

(i) ....

(ii)...

2 Standing or walking bent forwards, eyes on the ground

(i) ....

(ii)...

3 Sitting upright on the edge of a chair, hands tightly clenched

(i) ....

(ii)...

4 Sitting with hands and arms relaxed and legs slightly apart, maintaining eye contact with someone

(i) ....

(ii)...

5 Sitting with arms folded and legs crossed

(i) ....

(ii)...

This page may be photocopied for instructional use only. *The Dysfluency Resource Book* © J Turnbull & T Stewart 2010

Continued on Handout **12.2** ➜

6   Sitting slumped back in a chair, fiddling with the objects from your pocket (eg keys, money)

(i) ....

(ii)..

7   Sitting while the other person is standing

(i) ....

(ii)..

8   Standing while the other person is sitting

(i) ....

(ii)..

Routledge
Taylor & Francis Group

Observer checklist

Skill	Observed	Not observed
Kept appropriate eye contact		
Sat in appropriate position		
Looked relaxed and open		
Appeared interested, showed facial expression		
Did not interrupt or take the speaker's turn		
Used natural gestures as appropriate		
Did not fidget		
Used verbal prompts, eg 'mm', 'I see'		
Asked questions to clarify, if necessary		
Did not 'judge' or offer advice		
Did not take over the subject, maintained the speaker's topic		
Tolerated silence, if appropriate		

Routledge
Taylor & Francis Group

Story for listening exercise

A farmer in Lincolnshire had a corrugated iron roof put on his barn. Strong gales in the autumn blew the roof off and when the farmer found it two fields away it was twisted and mangled beyond repair.

A friend and lawyer advised him that the Ford Motor Company would pay him a good price for the scrap metal and the farmer decided to ship the roof to the company to see how much he could get for it. He crated it up in a very big wooden box and sent it off to Dagenham, marking it plainly with his return address so that the Ford Motor Company would know where to send the cheque.

Twelve weeks passed and the farmer didn't hear from Ford. Finally, he was on the verge of writing to them to find out what was the matter when he received a letter from them.

It said, 'We don't know what hit your car, mister, but we'll have it fixed by the fifteenth of next month'.

(Source unknown)

Routledge
Taylor & Francis Group

Checklist for listening exercise

	Volunteer 1	Volunteer 2	Volunteer 3	Volunteer 4	Volunteer 5
1 A farmer in Lincolnshire					
2 Corrugated iron roof on barn					
3 Strong gales in autumn blew roof off					
4 Found two fields away					
5 Twisted and mangled beyond repair					
6 A friend and lawyer					
7 Ford Motor Company					
8 Good price for scrap metal					
9 Crated it up in a very big wooden box					
10 Dagenham					
11 Marked plainly with return address					
12 Twelve weeks passed					
13 On verge of writing					
14 Received a letter					
15 We don't know what hit your car, mister					
16 Fixed by the fifteenth of next month					

Routledge

Listening skills observation exercise

During the week, observe people around you. Write an example of someone you see using each of the good or bad listening skills outlined in each box.

Someone who interrupts	Someone who is non-judgemental	Someone who does not check out information that is unclear	Someone who accepts what others say to them
Someone who avoids giving direct advice	Someone who does not attend fully to the speaker	Someone who gives direct advice	Someone who undervalues a person's problem by describing a worse event that happened to them
Someone who does not undervalue another person's problem	Someone who clarifies information when it is unclear	Someone who gives the speaker their full attention	Someone who does not interrupt
Someone who is not accepting of what another person says	Someone who gives the speaker the impression that there is time for them to talk	Someone who appears judgemental about another person's problem	Someone who fails to give the impression that there is time to talk

Routledge
Taylor & Francis Group

H16

Keeping the conversation going

Content involves what we say and how 'themes' pass from one person to another.
This can happen in one of three ways.

1 We mention similar thoughts and ideas about the topic under discussion, for example:

Person A: I've been looking at holiday brochures. Everything is so expensive. It's a bit of a
worry, but I don't want to let the family down.

Person B: Yes, it worries me too. I don't know how anyone finds the money.

2 We talk about a similar topic, but the information or the feelings we discuss are different,
for example:

Person A: I've been looking at holiday brochures. Everything is so expensive. It's a bit of a
worry, but I don't want to let the family down.

Person B: Yes, I have too. I've been saving up so it's not a problem for me.
or I don't have that worry. I don't enjoy holidays; I'd rather stay at home.

3 We maintain the same feelings, but change the topic. An example of this sort of content
is as follows:

Person A: I've been looking at holiday brochures. Everything is so expensive. It's a bit of a
worry, but I don't want to let the family down.

Person B: I've been looking at the price of an iPod. My son wants one for his birthday,
but I'm concerned I'll have to disappoint him.

3 | Information on stammering

Since we wrote the first edition of this book we have become aware that many of our clients now come to their first session far better informed about stammering than they were in the past. This is mainly due to the growth of information available on the internet, and in the UK especially, on the British Stammering Association's website www.stammering.org. The number of reasonably priced self-help books both on stammering and on mental health issues has also increased considerably.

Despite this, there are still some clients who arrive at the clinic having researched very little. They may, however, have been exposed to social myths and popular misconceptions about stammering or have watched television programmes on 'therapy' that claims to 'cure' stammering.

We would advise clinicians to start from the knowledge base of the client: to find out what he knows and doesn't know and then fill in the gaps as necessary. In our experience many clients are interested in knowing as much as possible about stammering. There are a number of key areas about which they may request information and clarification:

- the causes of stammering
- genetic/heredity factors
- personality and intelligence factors
- myths about stammering
- sex ratio
- incidence/prevalence data
- factors which may affect stammering, for example tiredness, stress, alcohol
- how others perceive stammering and a person who stammers
- treatments (including drug therapy, hypnotherapy, any current fads or trends and, increasingly, altered auditory feedback (AAF) devices)
- whether there is a cure.

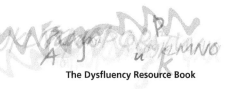
Activities *for providing information on non-fluency*

Handout 18 Basic information on stammering ℹ️ ⚙️

This handout can be given to a client early in therapy, sometimes after the first session. The client may be at the contemplation stage of change: well motivated to read the information in order to find out more about the nature and treatment of stammering and to use it to move into action. We suggest he comes back to the next session with any questions he may have. It is always interesting to see, at the second session, whether or not the handout has been read, what the client remembers of it, whether he has questions to ask, and if so, what they are. This can provide the clinician with much information about the client's readiness for change, the way he learns and his attitude to stammering.

Research ⚙️

An alternative method that we have used on occasions in group therapy is for clients to select an area of interest and carry out their own research on the topic. The results can then be presented to the group in a formal or an informal way and discussed.

Normal communication

Speech production

Along with many other clinicians we find it useful to give our clients information on how speech is normally produced. The philosophy behind this practice is that people need to know how their speech mechanisms ought to work in order to spot those aspects which are not functioning as they should.

When to use

This work is usually carried out relatively early on in therapy as the resulting increase in an individual's awareness is essential for the identification tasks that usually follow. However, clinicians must be aware that adults who stammer have often had several periods of therapy and some, if not all, of the details of speech production may not be new to them.

Teaching speech production

It is important that speech production is described in terms which are easily 'digestible' and that the process is demystified. One useful way of checking what clients actually know and then filling in any gaps is to ask them to fill in a questionnaire such as the one shown on Handout 19. In group therapy this can be worked on in pairs or small groups and the knowledge pooled. In one-to-one therapy it may be set as a home-based exercise and reviewed at a subsequent therapy session. In this case we ask clients not to research the subject at this stage but just to answer as best they can. Time can then be devoted to those aspects that were unclear or not understood.

We have structured the information on speech production into three main systems – respiration, phonation and articulation – as we believe these relate most closely to the processes that can break down during stammering.

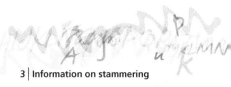

Respiration

In discussing respiration it is important to convey the following information:

- terminology

- muscular activity involved in inhalation and exhalation

- process of diaphragmatic breathing for speech

- some aspects of respiration that can cause difficulties in speech production (for example, speaking on exhaled air, reduced vital capacity).

Phonation

We consider the following to be important information concerning the process of phonation:

- terminology

- the part played by the larynx in speaking

- linguistic implications of laryngeal function (voiced and voiceless phonemes).

Articulation

The following information on articulation is included:

- terminology

- functions of articulators

- sound production, including place and manner

- discussion of minimal pairs.

Common problems

- A client still perceives he is being 'tested' and will fail. In a group setting, working in pairs or small groups can help. If the clinician judges that this sense of failure may be too great for a particular client, it may be best not to use the questionnaire but just to give a simple explanation of the processes involved.

- A client may worry that he will not understand the concepts involved. The clinician's role here is to give very clear and simple explanations.

- As for other aspects of identification, looking closely at speech can provoke anxiety. The clinician must always be on the lookout for such a reaction.

Activity for work on speech production

Questionnaire ⓘ ⚙

The questionnaire and answer sheet on Handouts 19 and 20 are examples that clinicians could use in therapy as they stand or as a basis for their own versions. On completion of this questionnaire the client is provided with a full set of answers and a diagram (Handout 21) to keep for future reference.

Basic information on stammering

NB The words 'stutter' and 'stammer' both mean the same. 'Stutter' is the word most commonly used in the USA and Australasia, while in the UK the word 'stammer' is more common.

How many people stammer?

- If you were to ask the population at large on any one occasion, approximately 1 per cent will report that they stammer. (You may see this referred to as *prevalence*.)

- The percentage of people who have ever stammered *at any time in their lives* (known as *incidence*) is generally considered to be around 5 per cent.

What sort of people stammer?

- In older children and adults more males stammer than females. The ratio is about 4:1. In young children the ratio is thought to be nearer to 2:1, suggesting that more girls than boys recover from stammering.

- There is no evidence to suggest that people who stammer are different (in any area other than speech) from people who do not stammer. For example, people who stammer are no more or less intelligent, extrovert, athletic, anxious and so on.

- A number of famous people stammer or have stammered in the past, which shows that there really is very little someone who stammers cannot do. The list includes:

  - heads of government/state: Winston Churchill, King George VI, Emperor Claudius

  - actors: Marilyn Monroe, James Earl Jones (the actor and voice of Darth Vader), Rowan Atkinson, Bruce Willis, Julia Roberts, Hugh Grant

  - singers: 'Scatman', Gareth Gates, Carly Simon

  - newsreaders and presenters: Martyn Lewis, Nicholas Parsons

  - writers: Lewis Carroll, Margaret Drabble

  - scientists: Steven Hawking, Charles Darwin

  - sportsperson: Tiger Woods

  - theatre director: Jonathan Miller

  - composer: Andrew Lloyd Webber

  - and even a spy!: Kim Philby.

When does stammering start?

- In children, non-fluent speech can occur as part of normal speech and language development. This can happen at any time from the beginning of talking up to five or six years of age. Sometimes it is difficult to differentiate this normal non-fluent speaking from stammering.

- Stammering itself most commonly begins between the ages of approximately two and five years, the average age being around three and a half. There are very few reported cases of stammering starting in adolescence.

Continued on Handout 18.2 →

- There is a tendency for children to recover spontaneously, although this likelihood decreases with age. More girls than boys recover.

- Sometimes stammering starts in adulthood, usually as a result of some sort of brain (neurological) problem such as a head injury or stroke. Occasionally, it is associated with a traumatic event or period of extreme stress. There were a number of cases of acquired stammering linked to 'shell shock' in World War 1.

Does stammering run in families?

- There is quite a lot of evidence to suggest that stammering can run in successive generations of the same family. One study estimated that the incidence of stammering among close relatives of those who stammer is more than three times that of the population as a whole.

- Research is ongoing to find specific genes that may be responsible for stammering.

- It also seems likely that heredity may play a part in whether someone will recover from stammering or whether their stammering will persist into adulthood.

- Heredity cannot be regarded as the whole story. There are several cases documented of identical twins reared apart where one stammered and one did not. This suggests that environmental factors must also play a part.

What causes stammering?

The short answer is that we do not yet know. However, research evidence over the last decade is leading us to believe that there is some difference in activity levels in the brains of people who stammer compared with those of fluent speakers. Some researchers have hypothesised that the difference may lie in the function of a part of the brain called the basal ganglia (Alm, 2004)[1].

Factors which often reduce stammering

- Speaking in an altered way. This includes using a different accent or voice, speaking more slowly, changing pitch, whispering and speaking in a monotone. Some people also report not stammering when on stage playing a role.

- Speaking at the same time as another person or group of people.

- Reading (for some people), perhaps because the words are already provided.

- Reading the same passage a few times. (This is sometimes called the 'adaptation effect'.)

- Saying something immediately after another person has said it.

- Speaking to small children and animals.

- Singing. We have very rarely met adults who stammer when singing. Singing requires continuous vibration of the vocal cords, controlled breathing and activity in a different part of the brain. It is also a more automatic behaviour, with an inbuilt rhythm that does not require the 'singer' to formulate what he has to sing (ie construct the sentences, choose the words, and so on). Most experts consider these differences as significant for maintaining fluent speech.

- Talking when alone or when feeling relaxed.

This page may be photocopied for instructional use only. *The Dysfluency Resource Book* © J Turnbull & T Stewart 2010

Routledge
Taylor & Francis Group

[1] 'Stuttering and the basal ganglia circuits', *Journal of Communication Disorders*, 37, pp325–69.

Continued on Handout **18.3** →

- Alcohol reduces stammering for some people. Perhaps it relaxes them.
- Distractors. Some people find that carrying out behaviours (such as tapping a pencil) while speaking helps them not think about their speech, and this seems to reduce stammering.

Factors which often make stammering worse

- Talking on the telephone.
- Talking in front of a group of people, especially if the speaker does not know them well.
- Being required to give specific information, for example name, address, date of birth.
- Speaking to authority figures.
- Reading (for some people) because they cannot easily avoid words.
- Stressful situations such as interviews.
- Alcohol (for some people, but see above). It maybe that alcohol takes away control over speech for this group of people.
- Increased emotion, for example, feeling anxious.

Treatments available for stammering

1 Speech and language therapy
This may include:

- psychological approaches such as counselling, personal construct psychology, cognitive behavioural therapy, solution-focused brief therapy
- desensitisation and avoidance reduction
- fluency-enhancing and stammering modification techniques
- relaxation and anxiety control
- assertiveness
- social and communication skills training.

2 Hypnotherapy

3 Drug therapy
Some family doctors prescribe tranquillisers for adults who stammer as a short-term treatment.

4 Psychotherapy

5 Altered auditory feedback (AAF) devices
In recent years a number of devices have come on to the market for people who stammer which change the feedback or the sound of their speech which they hear. These devices are worn in either one or both ears and enable people to hear their own speech but with a slight delay and with a change of pitch (ie either a lower or higher sounding voice).

6 Other
From time to time 'independent' individuals will advertise courses, usually for adult stammerers, although increasingly these are including children. These courses are often based

This page may be photocopied for instructional use only. *The Dysfluency Resource Book* © J Turnbull & T Stewart 2010

on their own experience of stammering and their own 'cure'. These courses tend to use the same approach for all clients.

Society's view of stammering

In the course of our group therapy programmes, clients have surveyed views on stammering in Leeds (further described in Chapter 7 'Desensitisation'). We continue to be surprised by the suggested causes of stammering. Some of the less informed responses suggest it is caused by:

- anxiety or 'nerves'
- a physical cause, such as 'short tongue' or brain damage
- imitation of another person who stammers (usually in childhood)
- consuming hot and/or cold food or drinks
- lack of religious faith and prayer.

Is there a cure?

The short answer is 'no'. However, it is well documented that it is very easy to increase an adult's level of fluency with a direct, intensive approach within a short space of time. (Our experience has been of dramatic improvements in 80 per cent of clients over a weekend!) The research and our practice also show that such rapid improvement is generally not well maintained and fluency frequently breaks down within a matter of months. For changes to be meaningful and maintained over a period of some years our recommendation is that change is made slowly and at the client's pace.

Routledge
Taylor & Francis Group

Normal speech production: questionnaire

This questionnaire is designed to help you find out what you know about how speech is produced – not something most people normally think about. It is not a test! Your answers will be used to help your therapist fill in any gaps in your understanding.

Understanding the 'normal' speech mechanism can help you to understand what might be happening when things go wrong with your own speaking.

Breathing

1 Another name for breathing is ....

2 Breathing has two phases. What are they called?...

3 Put your hands flat on your lower ribs with the fingers meeting at the breastbone.
   Breathe in. What happens to your fingers? ....

4 Breathe out. What is happening now? ....

   ....

5 While you are talking, are you breathing out or in? ....

6 If you only fill part of your lungs when you breathe in, what problems might this create?

   ....

7 Try to keep speaking without a breath: what happens? ....

   ....

   ....

Making sound (in the throat)

1 What do you call the place (organ) where you produce sound?...

2 What do the vocal cords do? ....

   ....

3 Say the words 'Sue' and 'zoo' several times slowly. What do you notice about the difference
   between the 's' and 'z' sounds? (Clue: try putting your finger on your Adam's apple.)

   ....

   ....

This page may be photocopied for instructional use only. *The Dysfluency Resource Book* © J Turnbull & T Stewart 2010

Routledge
Taylor & Francis Group

Continued on Handout **19.2** ➜

4 Can you find any other pairs of sounds that behave in the same way as 's' and 'z'?

....

....

Articulation (making sounds in the mouth)

1 Which parts of your mouth do you use to make sounds? ....

....

2 The letters of the alphabet can be divided into two main categories. What are they?

....

3 What is the difference in the way these two kinds of sounds are made? ....

....

....

....

4 Name one or more sounds you make by:

(a) putting your lips together ....

(b) putting your top teeth over your bottom lip ....

(c) putting your tongue tip behind your teeth and letting it go. ....

5 Say 't' and then say 's'. Can you identify one main difference between them in the way they are made?

....

....

....

....

6 What parts of your mouth are involved in making the sounds (i) 'k' and (ii) 'm'?

....

....

Routledge
Taylor & Francis Group

Normal speech production: answers to questionnaire

Breathing

1 Respiration

2 Inhalation/inspiration, exhalation/expiration

3 They are pushed outwards and upwards

4 Your fingers return to the original position: they move inwards and downwards

5 Out

6 Running out of air frequently, poor phrasing, low volume, tense posture

7 The sound becomes quieter until it stops altogether, the voice becomes more and more strained and the pitch of the voice may rise. You get more and more tense

Making sound

1 Voice box or larynx

2 They vibrate when air is forced between them, causing a sound to be made

3 The vocal cords vibrate and produce sound for 'z' and not for 's'. 'S' is known as a voiceless sound and 'z' as a voiced sound for that reason

4 p and b, t and d, k and g, f and v, ch and j. There are others but they are hard to write down!

Articulation

1 Lips, teeth, roof of the mouth (hard/soft palate), tongue

2 Vowels and consonants

3 Vowels are made through a free opening of the mouth and are not stopped by the organs of articulation. In consonants some kind of obstruction is made to the free passage of sound

4 (i) p, b, m
   (ii) f, v
   (iii) t, d

5 There is a different way of producing the sound: 't' produced quickly following a build-up of air pressure in the mouth, 's' produced by air being forced through a narrowing in the mouth

6 (i) tongue, soft palate (lower jaw)
   (ii) lips (nose)

Routledge

Speech production

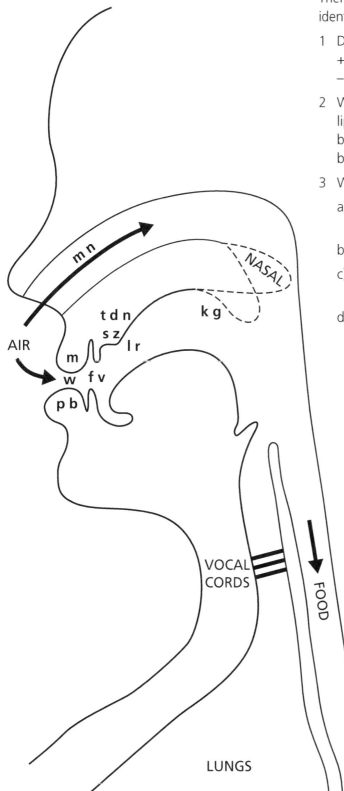

There are 3 main points that we can use to identify the character of a sound:

1 Does it have VOICE or not?
   + voice: **vowels, d, g, m, l, z, v**
   – voice: **s, f, p, k**

2 Where is the main place of articulation?
   lips: **p, b, m, w**
   behind teeth: **t, d, s, z, n**
   back: **k, g**

3 What is happening to the airstream?

   a) stopped altogether = PLOSIVE/STOP
      p, b, t, d, k, g

   b) squeezed = FRICATIVE **s, z, f, v, th, sh**

   c) air passing freely through nose =
      NASAL **m, n**

   d) airstream not obstructed =
      CONTINUOUS **r, l, w, y, vowels**

Routledge
Taylor & Francis Group

4 | Variation: non-speech and speech

In discussing variation, Van Riper (1973) writes that the 'hallmark' of variation experiments is change. The aim of variation is to give an adult who stammers a sense of choice. He does not have to behave in the way he behaves, nor indeed stammer in the manner he does, but can choose another pattern of behaviour. It may be that he has progressively reduced the choices he has in his life until he is at the point when he sees no other options but the routine types of behaviour in which he is currently engaged. Many adults we have met talk vehemently about not being able to fulfil their potential and having choice taken away from them because of their speech difficulties. In fact, many have 'imprisoned' themselves as a way of hiding from and concealing their stammer. This does not have to be so. As Kelly (1991) says, individuals do not have to be a product of their own biography. Variation is a process that can enable adults who stammer to realise this.

The foundation of recent work on variation, in the UK at least, owes much to the influence of personal construct psychology.

When to use

Variation activities are best used at the beginning of therapy:

• before work on fluency techniques

• alongside work on identification.

How to use

In this approach, which we described earlier (see Chapter 1), a client is encouraged to 'loosen' his system of construing by experimenting with:

• different ways of behaving

• different ways of feeling

• different ways of thinking.

The person can choose subsequently to accept, reject or modify these options, but the experiment will have illustrated that he has a choice. Change is introduced in as unthreatening a way as possible.

Stage 1. An individual is asked to change some aspect of his life that he sees as relatively unimportant to him (for example, related to his appearance or any routines he may have). Following the experiment the client reports back specifically on how the change was made, whether it was easy or difficult to implement, how he felt making it and whether other people noticed and/or commented on the difference.

Stage 2. After these experiments on more peripheral behaviours, therapy moves slowly into varying features of communication, for example:

• use of gestures

• facial expression

• initiating conversation.

Stage 3. Finally, the client is asked to change specific speech behaviours. (Moving to the variation of speech behaviours has direct links with the first stages of block modification and, ideally, the client can move seamlessly from one to another without realising it. For example, he can move on from varying speech behaviours to identifying and changing his own stammering.) Once again, it is suggested that the individual begins in a less threatening way, by experimenting with speech changes that are unrelated to the way he stammers, for example:

• tone of voice

• volume

• intonation.

Later, work on stammering behaviours is introduced. Van Riper (1973) recommends targeting what he calls 'anticipatory' behaviours, such as postponement and avoidance, as he has found these are more easily varied and more under the person's control. Through applying principles from behavioural psychology, the stereotypical, habitual pattern of stammering is disrupted. This can be done in a variety of ways:

• adding to the stammering by inserting another type of behaviour

• changing (the behaviour itself or the order in which it occurs)

• diminishing it or removing it altogether

• contrasting it with another behaviour.

Examples of these changes can be found in the activities section that follows.
In our experience we have noted that change at this point can be quite dramatic, with clients reporting, for example, a marked increase in their fluency and feelings of control when experimenting with reducing 'backtracking'.

Common problems

Resistance. As clinicians we can observe those 'important' aspects in our clients and become more aware perhaps of those individuals who are resistant to even minor change and find it very difficult to implement. In situations where change is more difficult the implications are clear for the therapist and the client himself: how will he react to change which is much more fundamental, that is, change to his speech, which has been a part of him and his self-image for several decades? Also, therapy will have to take into account the client's need to feel in control and to feel that he can make his own decisions.

Significant others. Sometimes difficulties arise from significant others in clients' lives. A wife or girlfriend may dislike fundamental changes in her partner's role that impact on their relationship. In these instances we need to engage important others and help them understand the processes the client is engaged in if change is to be achieved.

Problems with varying stammering. In attempting to reduce some of the more covert strategies used to hide stammering, some clients lose the little fluency they enjoy and feel that their speech is even more out of control than previously. (This is discussed in greater detail in Chapter 7 'Desensitisation'.)

Timing. A final point to be made here is about the insight that variation experiments can give to the clinician. They can reveal much about how easy or difficult an individual finds change. Undoubtedly, there are some clients for whom change of any sort is very stressful, but they have reached a point in their lives when they have had enough of limited choices and restricted life styles. For these individuals, variation remains threatening, but the option of holding on to the status quo is much less attractive and therefore they will attempt the change. For others, the threat that change brings is too great and staying the same is safer. We recommend that for these clients variation is taken at a much slower pace and for a longer time. If the client remains resistant, then perhaps consideration should be given to whether or not therapy at this time is appropriate (see the section 'The stages of change' in Chapter 1 'Principles of therapy'). Proceeding with speech modification in the absence of loosening and/ or variation is foolhardy and cannot be justified. For some individuals, it may just not be the right time to change and variation experiments can help determine this.

Activities for non-speech variation

Talking about change 🛈 ⚙

The following discussion topics are useful preparatory activities that can be carried out in a group or individual therapy setting.

Decision making
Each client talks about decisions that he:

• might have made

• wishes he had made

• is glad were not made.

Significant life-turning events
Each client discusses his history in terms of significant points in his life. The clinician(s) and/or group members should be encouraged to pinpoint why these events were significant and what influenced the change in direction in thinking, attitude and/or behaviour.

How changes are made
Each client recounts an event or situation in which he was required to make a choice, for example, applying for a job, getting married, moving house. The discussion should centre on how the decision to change was brought about, how the individual made a decision and what factors affected the final choice.

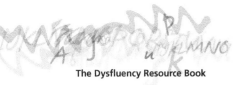
Experiments that create choice ⓘ ⚙ [1]

In the first instance, an individual is asked to change some peripheral aspect of his life. This might be related to:

- appearance (for example, wearing/not wearing jewellery, growing/shaving off a beard or moustache)

- routines (for example, the route taken to work, the daily newspaper which is bought or the types of sandwiches/food eaten for lunch)

- life style (for example, trying different exercise regimes, slowing down the pace of life, getting up/going to bed at different times or becoming involved in household chores not previously carried out).

Applying guidelines ⓘ ⚙

Handout 22 'Guidelines for experimenting with change' can be discussed with an individual client or presented to a group for discussion. Alternatively, clinicians may use it as an example on which to base their own version.

Evaluation after experimentation ⓘ ⚙

The following questions could be used as the basis of a discussion with the client(s) after the experiment:

What exactly was the experiment?

Were other people informed?

How did you tell them? *or*

Why did you choose not to tell them?

What do you think about your decision to tell/not to tell others now?

What did you predict would happen?

What did you predict you would feel?

What did you predict you would think?

Did you believe the experiment was achievable?

What aspects of the experiment were achieved?

How did you feel before, during and after the experiment?

What did you think before, during and after the experiment?

How did other people respond?

Did anything surprise you?

What did you learn?

Is the experiment worth continuing?

If you were to do it again, what would you keep the same?

If you were to do it again, what would you do differently?

---

[1] These experiments can be carried out as part of an individual therapy programme, but the best results are often achieved in a group setting. In this context a client is encouraged to make changes by fellow clients, rather than by 'fluent' therapists, he receives much encouragement for his efforts and is often motivated by the steps taken by others. In addition, pressure can be brought to bear by peers rather than therapists, and this can be a major factor for change.

Activities for communication and speech variation

Communication ⓘ 🄖

As in non-speech variation, the client is encouraged to experiment first with changing aspects of his general communication skills that pose less of a threat. Some examples are given below; however, clinicians should discuss the options with the client and encourage him to make the choice.

Gesture

Increase the amount of hand/arm gesturing during one conversation a day.

Reduce/eliminate hand movements whenever you describe an event, situation or task.

Make a note of another person's use of gesture and (if appropriate) imitate one of their typical gestures.

Facial expression

For 10 minutes every day try to show others what you are feeling by increasing your facial expression.

Smile more.

Keep looking at people when they talk to you.

Encourage people when they speak to you by using facial expression.

Observe the faces of 10 people you talk to every day.

Eye contact

Maintain eye contact with everyone who talks to you.

Work on keeping eye contact during your biggest stammers. Start by focusing on this for one particular hour each day.

Find out when your partner loses eye contact with you when they are:

• talking

• listening to you talk.

Find out when you look away from other people who are talking to you.

Find out when you look away from other people when you are talking to them.

Pausing

Insert a short (two-second) pause before you answer other people's questions.

Insert a 'thinking pause' into seven conversations each day.

Observe how long you can wait before answering someone's question.

Observe which of your friends uses the most pauses in their speech.

Try pausing at the end of sentences (that is, where you would expect to see a full stop if the sentence was written down) before proceeding on to the next sentence. Use this in a conversation where you have lots to say.

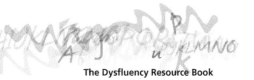
Pragmatics

Ask as many questions as you can of your colleagues while at work.

Talk to one new person each day (for example, say 'hello' to the cleaner or caretaker, talk to someone at the bus stop or on the train, greet someone in the lift and say something about the weather).

Say an extra sentence when buying your regular newspaper, lunchtime sandwich or bus ticket.

At the beginning of the day find out how other people have spent their evenings or weekends.

Make a point of having lunch with a colleague each working day and engaging them in conversation.

Tell one other person one thing about yourself each day.

Ask one other person one thing about themselves each day.

Speech variation ⓘ ⚙ [2]

Experiment first with varying features of speech which are not directly associated with stammering behaviours. The following are examples of tasks that could be used. (See also Handout 23 'Experimenting with your speech'.)

Volume

Try slightly increasing the volume of your voice when talking to people at work. (The increased volume must be slight but noticeable.)

Use a louder voice for the first hour in the morning and a quieter voice at the end of the day.

Concentrate on not allowing the volume of your voice to fade at the end of sentences or towards the end of what you have to say.

Use a quieter voice with (your) children and/or pets.

Be aware of varying the volume of your speech in the same conversation, to convey emotion (for example, excitement vs sadness or disappointment).

Speed

Increase the speed of your speech when you feel relaxed.

Gradually increase the speed of your speech towards the end of sentences or the end of an utterance.

Slow down your speech when you talk to your boss or someone you think of as important.

Experiment with varying the rate of your speech: have two 'faster' hours followed by two 'slower' hours.

Read to your children or partner using a faster and then a slower speed. Ask them which they prefer.

---

[2] Note that these tasks varying speech behaviours can flow easily from other more general variation experiments.

Intonation and stress

Experiment with giving the first word of a sentence more emphasis.

Try and make your voice more interesting (that is, where your voice would naturally rise, let it rise slightly more and, similarly, where your voice would naturally fall, let it fall a little further). Use this way of speaking when reading to your partner or children once a day.

Use a 'softer' approach by keeping the number of words you emphasise to a minimum.

For the first hour of the day use a flat voice, with little or no change in tone.

Varying stammering behaviour ⓘ ⚙

A client can change the way he stammers in a variety of ways. The principles of varying stammering behaviours are:

1 add

2 diminish/remove

3 change

4 contrast.

These can be applied to most stammering behaviours, as in the following examples.

1 Reduce backtracking using addition, such as 'It's my turn, it's my turn, it's my turn now'. Whenever the client is aware of backtracking he must add another element of the backtracking to the utterance: It's my turn, it's my turn, it's my turn, *it's my* turn now'.

2 Work on prolongations using diminishing, such as 'It's myyyyyyyyyy turn now'. Whenever the client is aware (or reminded) that he is prolonging a vowel he has to shorten the prolongation: 'It's myyyyy turn now'.

    Removing a behaviour can also be used in the context of fillers. For example, a client who uses 'You know' or 'You know what I mean' could be encouraged to try to cut this out of his speech for a week to see the effect it has. This can be quite difficult to do initially and may need lots of practice and small intermediate steps.

3 Repetitions may be varied by changing them into prolongations. For example, if a person repeats the first syllable of a word, he should be encouraged to extend one of the repetitions. Thus 'tu, tu, tu, turn' becomes 'tu, tu, tuuuurn'. This can be modelled by the clinician and shadowed (said simultaneously with him) as the client speaks.

    Similarly, 'ers' could be changed to 'ums' for an experimental period.

4 Eliminating accessory movements such as foot tapping can be achieved effectively by using a contrasting behaviour (for example, finger tapping.) So, whenever the client taps his foot, he must tap his finger too.

Further specific examples can be found in Chapter 7 'Desensitisation' and Chapter 9 'Avoidance reduction therapy'.

Guidelines for experimenting with change

The purpose of experimentation is to test out a hypothesis, for example, 'It is better for me to do x than y'. In an experiment you are choosing to do something differently in order to experience the difference and gather data. As a result of the experience you are able to validate or disprove your hypothesis for that particular event: 'Yes, it is better to do x' or 'No, y is better'.

- Choose something that will be noticed by others.

- Choose something that feels achievable, even in the short term.

  Remember this is only an experiment; it does not have to be something that is irreversible. You can choose.

- Choose something that is about you and/or the way you live your life, but something that is not too important to you.

- Choose whether or not to tell other people what you are doing.

  In some instances it may be better to prepare others in advance so that they will create the 'space' for you to experiment, for example, doing household chores normally carried out by your partner. In other cases it may be preferable not to inform other people so that you can observe their reactions to the change more objectively.

- Treat the variation as if it were an actual experiment. Work out a hypothesis, for example: 'I am going to get up early every day for a week to see if getting to work on time is easier and makes me more productive at work.' Predict what you think will happen, for example, 'I am not going to find this easy. I will be grumpy in the morning, miss the extra sleep and be more tired at the end of the day.'

- Carry out the experiment as specified and record what happens. For example, make a note of how you felt on day one when the alarm went off, what your feelings were and the reactions of others when you arrived early at work. Then at the end of the day record whether you felt more tired as you had predicted. Be sure to register your feelings as well as the actual results of the variation.

Routledge
Taylor & Francis Group

Experimenting with your speech

Having experimented with doing some things differently in your daily life, it is now time to experiment with your speech. Once again you are invited to consider testing a hypothesis, this time about talking. This experiment will help you develop different ways of thinking and feeling as well as different ways of talking.

Stage 1. Start with an aspect of your communication that is not too difficult to change. Choose from one of the following.

Volume of your speech

Here are some examples you could try out.

Try slightly increasing the volume of your voice when talking to people at work. (The increased volume must be slight but noticeable.)

Use a louder voice for the first hour in the morning and a quieter voice at the end of the day.

Concentrate on not allowing the volume of your voice to fade at the end of sentences or towards the end of what you have to say.

Use a quieter voice with (your) children and/or pets.

Be aware of varying the volume of your speech in the same conversation, to convey emotion (for example, excitement vs sadness or disappointment).

Tone and expression of your speech

Experiment with giving the first word of a sentence more emphasis.

Try and make your voice more interesting (that is, where your voice would naturally rise, let it rise slightly more and, similarly, where your voice would naturally fall, let it fall a little further). Use this way of speaking when reading to your partner or children once a day.

Use a 'softer' approach by keeping the number of words you emphasise to a minimum.

For the first hour of the day use a flat voice, with little or no change in tone.

Speed of your speech

Increase the speed of your speech when you feel relaxed.

Gradually increase the speed of your speech towards the end of sentences or at the end of an utterance.

Slow down your speech when you talk to your boss or someone you think of as important.

Experiment with varying the rate of your speech: have two 'faster' hours followed by two 'slower' hours.

Read to your children or partner using a faster and then a slower speed. Ask them which they prefer.

This page may be photocopied for instructional use only. *The Dysfluency Resource Book* © J Turnbull & T Stewart 2010

Continued on Handout **23.2** →

Stage 2. Now look at ways of varying your stammering. Choose from one of the following.

Add

If you use 'run-ins' or 'backtracking' an experiment could involve adding some of these types of speech. For example, 'It's my turn, it's my turn, it's my turn now' would become' 'It's my turn, it's my turn, it's my turn, *it's my* turn now'.

Diminish

If you have stretches or prolongations as part of your stammer, try experimenting with shortening or reducing their length. For example, 'It's myyyyyyyyy turn now' would become 'It's myyyyy turn now'.

Remove

This is a useful technique to experiment with if you use lots of fillers such as 'you know' and 'actually'. For example, 'you know' or 'you know what I mean' could be targeted. If you count five in one conversation, try to reduce it to three or four in the next conversation, then one or two in the next.

Change

Types of stammering can also be varied. For example, if you repeat the first sound of a word, try to turn the last one into a stretched or prolonged sound. For example, 'tu, tu, tu, turn' becomes 'tu, tu, tuuuurn'. Similarly, 'ers' could be changed to 'ums' for the length of a conversation or for an hour during the day.

Contrast

Getting rid of extra movements such as foot tapping can be achieved effectively by using a contrasting movement such as tapping your finger. So, whenever you tap your foot, you must tap your finger at the same time.

Routledge

5 | Identification

Identification is the process by which a person comes to an understanding that his stammer is made up of various components and develops an ability to recognise, name and monitor these features. However, by engaging in such an activity the individual is also directly confronting his difficulties and the fear associated with them. This can be the first time he has chosen to do this, maybe after a lifetime of running away or trying to hide specific behaviours or feelings from himself and others. As such, the process of identification can provide the foundation and, as Manning writes, 'some distance and objectivity' (2000, p282) for work on desensitisation and avoidance reduction.

Identification may first have been advocated by members of the Iowa movement in the 1930s. Bryngelson recommended that an individual should try to replicate his stammering by observing himself closely in a mirror. Van Riper (1973) also used identification as the basis for his block modification techniques (see Chapter 14 'Block modification').

When to use

When discussing the treatment of stammering, Van Riper (1973) argues that it is important to start therapy with identification as this avoids placing too much demand on a client to immediately modify his speech. However, our experience has shown that for some clients this process can bring about the realisation that there is a lot to change.

We recommend identification be used with all clients. We suggest identification activities are carried out alongside 'loosening' of construing, as discussed in Chapter 1, and after the client has been given general background information on speech and language terminology, stammering and so on.

Teaching identification

Van Riper uses a hierarchy in identification therapy that appears to be linked to a time line or sequence of events in terms of how a stammering episode might occur.

The behaviours associated with 'before' stammering. Van Riper lists these as fluent stuttering, avoidance behaviours, postponement, timing or starting devices.

The stammering episode itself. Van Riper includes under this section verbal cues that signal stammering, situational cues, core stammering behaviours, tension and repetitive recoil.

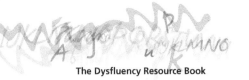
The identification of post-stammering reactions. In this final stage Van Riper includes frustration, shame and feelings of hostility.

Most clinicians, certainly in the UK, divide identification into work first on the overt features and then on covert aspects of stammering. We consider the overt characteristics to be a little less threatening for most clients and therefore easier to start to consider and discuss.

Overt symptoms

The overt characteristics of stammering are those that could be noticeable to people if they are really good observers and/or listeners. We would include under this category specific types of stammering behaviour:

- repetitions
- silent or audible prolongations
- disrupted breathing patterns
- loci of tension
- secondary body movements
- unhelpful non-verbal behaviour (including consideration of eye contact, facial expression, posture)
- rate of speech
- other problematic vocal and/or verbal aspects of communication (such as voice quality, pitch, volume, pragmatic abilities and so on).

Indeed, it is impossible to list all the possible overt features because of the individual and variable nature of stammering.

In therapy there should be some agreement as to which labels will be used, and clinicians are recommended to use the same terms as their clients as this increases understanding and meaning for the client. Some clients prefer to use certain words for their difficulty, for example, 'speech defect' rather than 'stammer', as this is less challenging or more acceptable to them. Later, as part of a desensitisation process, this can be challenged, but at this stage it is important to accept the client's terminology.

Common problems

Van Riper was of the opinion that people who stammer are not aware of what they do when they stammer.

> One of the curious features in the stutterer's perception of his stuttering is his tendency to lump together a host of disparate behaviors ranging all the way from nose wrinkling to saying 'ah-ah-ah' and to call that lump stuttering. When you ask him what he did, he will merely tell you that he stuttered.
> (1973, p246)

Thus, the main issue when working on identification is increasing a client's monitoring of his own behaviour at a level of detail that will facilitate change. Some clients find it very difficult to identify what they do. As a result, clinicians will need to draw on a variety of different

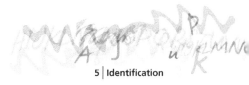
media – audio, visual, tactile and kinaesthetic feedback – to enable clients to recognise what they are doing during stammering. Another issue is getting clients to accept clinicians' and others' feedback on their stammering behaviour. Having other individuals who stammer and/ or significant others give feedback rather than a clinician can increase the value the individual client places on the feedback he is receiving. Due to clients' sensitivity about their stammering, the process of identification needs to progress at an appropriate pace for them to come to terms with and 'own' their stammering behaviours.

Therapy for overt identification

Identification can be used within both individual therapy and group therapy regimes. In one-to-one sessions it has been found useful to move the client slowly towards full identification of his problem. Manning stresses the importance of the client listing and writing down his stammering features. In this way he is 'assuming responsibility for this behaviour' (2000, p282). A useful process can be summarised as follows:

- Consider features that the client is aware of – what he notices or recognises in his own speech – and examine these aspects first in some depth.

- Gradually draw his attention to other behaviours about which he has no awareness, using the same depth of analysis.

- Use audio, DVD or video recording late in the process. In our experience, feedback of this type can be a challenge to the individual to confront his stammering head on and he may not be ready to do this.

In groups, clients can provide valuable insights into each other's stammering, which can, in turn, help them identify similar features in their own speech. Working in small groups or in pairs is a little less threatening. We advocate a similar process to the one described above, starting from the client's own perceptions and then gradually introducing additional features to be analysed.

Activities for overt identification

Brainstorm overt features ⓘ ✿
Brainstorm all possible stammering behaviours. Compare the list generated by clients with Handout 24 'Describing overt stammering symptoms'.

Describing overt stammering symptoms ⓘ ✿
Give out Handout 24 'Describing overt stammering symptoms' and discuss its relevance to the client(s).

Observation ✿
In pairs, one person talks to their partner about a selected topic, such as their leisure pursuits, work, family. Then they reverse roles. Using Table 5.1 'Checklist for monitoring overt stammering', they should note all the overt stammering features they observe in the other person during the task and feed this information back to the full group. If time and group numbers allow, it is useful to have each group member speak to and observe every other

group member. In this way the information is likely to cover a number of different aspects and, where several members mention one aspect of behaviour, this is given greater recognition and its importance is underlined.

Table 5.1 Checklist for monitoring overt stammering

Overt stammering	Description: What, when, how?	Frequency count: How many in a minute?
Sound/syllable/word/phrase repetitions		
Silent/audible prolongations		
Blocks		
Added extras, eg starters, fillers, 'ers'/'ums'		
Hard attacks		
Body movements		
Disrupted breathing patterns		
Rate problems		
Tension: – in stomach – in chest/shoulders – in throat/voice box – in mouth/jaw		

Checklist of overt stammering behaviours ⓘ ⚙

A client completes a checklist, initially on his own or alongside the clinician. His perceptions can be compared or checked either with the clinician in the case of individual therapy, or with other group members in a group programme. We recommend that time is spent on each individual checklist and clients should not be given several checklists together in one session. For example, we usually start with the overt checklist (Handout 25), followed by the covert and, finally, the avoidance checklist (Handouts 28 and 31 in Chapter 6 'Covert identification').

Home-based observation exercises

Based on the previous observation exercise, a number of tasks can be set for completion before the next group or individual session.

The client observes himself speaking in one situation every day (a different situation each day, if possible) and looks for overt stammering features under one or more categories mentioned by the group and/or clinician, or from the monitoring table.

In addition to or in place of self-observation, the client asks a 'significant other' person to use the monitoring sheet and point out overt features of his stammer when he talks to them. He may need to direct them to key categories such as breathing, rate and so on.

Using the monitoring sheets that other group members or the clinician have completed, the client makes a note of the overt features that he did not realise he employed. He should use these as a basis for an observation task to see if these features occur in other situations outside the group.

Describing overt stammering symptoms

Repetitions

Repetitions can occur:

- on sounds usually at the beginning of words, eg 'c, c, can', or occasionally at the end of words as in 'can n, n, n', or, rarely, in the middle: 'ca, a, a, n'

- on syllables either at the beginning of words, eg 'hip, hip, hippopotamus', or sometimes in the middle as in 'hippo, pot, pot, potamus'

- on whole words, eg 'in, in, in the country'

- on groups of words or phrases, eg 'I want, I want, I want coffee', or 'Try to, try to, try to find the answer'.

Silent and/or audible prolongations

Prolongations can be:

- stretched vowels, eg ooooooooooon top or tooooooooooooo

- consonants, eg sssssssssssssssspeech.

It would be unusual for the prolongation always to occur on a particular sound, for example on every 's' that occurred in a sentence. The sound feels as if it is 'stuck' in the mouth, throat or chest and this can last for several seconds.

Prolongation can also be caused by:

- the 'freezing' of speech muscles while trying to make sounds, which can sound like extended silences to a listener. These are sometimes called 'blocks'.

Extra or associated behaviours

Fillers. Adding in extra sounds or words when talking. This may be a way of gaining time or enabling the person to start speaking.

For example:

- adding sounds before certain words or sounds that are perceived as difficult to say, eg 'n, n, Leeds', 'l, l, Newcastle'

- adding sounds or words to help start a sentence, such as 'actually' as in 'Actually, I would like to eat a curry', or phrases such as 'you know', eg 'You know, I would like to eat a curry'; these are known as 'starters'

- using other non-speech sounds when speaking, eg coughing, throat clearing

- using 'ers' and 'ums' to excess, eg 'Er, I would, em, like, er, to eat, er, a curry'.

Word substitution. Changing or switching a word for another with an associated meaning, eg 'I would like to eat a, something hot and spicy'.

Circumlocution. Changing a sentence or a phrase around to make it easier to say, or talking around a topic to work up to saying a particularly difficult word, eg 'The last time I went to …, I used to go to Durham quite a lot and when I went on Tuesday …'.

Hard attack

When someone forces out a sound or word, the muscles and parts of the mouth that are used to make sound (eg lips, tongue) can become tense and tight. In addition, the air can be pushed out and the whole utterance will appear rushed and with a strained quality. This is called hard attack.
The opposite and preferred method of producing speech is soft contact, where the articulators (the parts of the mouth used in speech) move together gently, the breath is exhaled in a relaxed way and the sound is not forced or rushed.

Routledge
Taylor & Francis Group

Continued on Handout **24.2** →

Body movements during speech

Sometimes people develop body movements or 'accessory behaviours' alongside stammering. These movements may initially help to reduce the stammer or help the individual get through a difficult episode. However, in time they lose their effectiveness but remain fixed with the stammering. Here are a number of such movements:

- fidgeting
- excessive movements of arms or legs
- frequent changes of posture
- fiddling with hands, fingers or an object such as a pen
- clenching hands
- covering face, eyes, mouth
- touching hair, head
- jerking or moving head to one side
- tapping feet or fingers (perhaps to develop a rhythm to speak along with).

Disrupted breathing patterns

Breathing can be disrupted in a number of ways:

- Breathing in may be rushed, too frequent, too shallow and/or the breath may be too deep or tense.
- Breathing out may not be gradual: too much air may be released at the beginning of an utterance or exhalation may appear tense.
- Speech and breathing may be uncoordinated: ie the individual may try to speak either while breathing in or when running out of air.

Rate problems

There is a common myth that stammering is the result of speaking too quickly. In fact, there are a number of rate problems that can be associated with stammering:

fast speed: speeding up with greater fluency, speeding up immediately after stammering

slow speech: slowing down before anticipating stammering

problems with pausing: finding it hard to pause, making too few pauses in speech, pausing for too long.

Tension

A person may experience tension during speech and also when leading up to or after stammering. This may be:

- all over the body
- in the head (increased pressure)
- in the face (forehead, jaw)
- in the speech muscles (tongue, lips)
- in the neck and shoulders
- in the throat (where the voice box is)
- in the stomach and chest
- in the arms and legs.

Routledge
Taylor & Francis Group

Checklist of overt stammering behaviours

Consider which of the following features are part of your stammer. Tick all those you think apply to you, answer the questions about the features that are relevant to you and jot some notes down about them. Your clinician will be interested in any observations you make.

Repetitions

Which of these do you do? Tick those that are appropriate:

- sounds, eg 'c, c, can' or perhaps 'can, n, n'
- syllables or parts of words, eg 're, re, repetitions' or 'repeti, ti, tions'
- words, eg 'on, on, on Sunday'
- phrases, eg 'I want, I want, I want to buy this' or 'Go back, go back'

How are these repetitions produced?

- hurried, in bursts which appear out of control
- tense and forced out
- easy, unhurried

How long do they last, on average?

- a second or two
- several seconds
- longer than several seconds

Do these repetitions happen at any particular time, such as when you are relaxed, when you are under pressure, or at the end of the day? List some situations or occasions when you notice repetitions occurring.

....

....

....

....

Prolongations and blocks

Do you prolong (stretch out) or get stuck on any of these sounds? Tick the ones that apply:

- vowels: a, e, i o u
- consonants: can you list any particular ones?

How are your prolongations produced?

- no sound comes out
- the sound gets stuck in my chest
- the sound gets stuck in my throat
- the sound gets stuck in my mouth
- the sound gets stuck ....

.... (fill in the blank)

How long does the sound or block typically last?

- a second or two
- several seconds
- longer than several seconds

Do these prolongations happen at any particular time, such as when you are more relaxed, when you are under pressure, or at the end of the day? List some situations or occasions when you notice prolongations occurring.

....

....

....

....

....

Routledge

Continued on Handout **25.2** ➜

'Extras' when talking

Do you add in extra sounds or words when you talk? (These may be devices to give you more time or perhaps to get you started.) Do you:

- add sounds before certain words or sounds you think may be difficult to say, eg 'n, n, Jackie', 'l, l, Trudy'
- add sounds/words/phrases, eg 'actually', 'you know', to help you get started
- use other non-speech sounds when speaking, eg coughing, throat clearing, sniffs
- use 'ers' and 'ums' to excess
- other?

Do you have little tricks to help you talk that other people might see or hear? (Later we will consider ones that only you are aware of.) Do you:

- change a word
- change a sentence or a phrase around to make it easier to say
- take a long time to make your point
- not join in conversations
- pretend you have forgotten
- pretend to think
- other? Please list.

....

....

....

....

....

....

General features of communication

1 *Volume*

- Do you tend to speak too loudly or too quietly in some or all situations?
- Does your volume vary appropriately to match the situation?
- Is the volume of your speech affected by your stammering?

2 *Pitch*

- Is the pitch of your voice generally too high or too low?
- Does your voice lack variety of tone and appear flat and monotonous?
- Is the pitch of your speech affected by your stammering?

3 *Speed*

- Is the speed of your speech too quick or too slow?
- Do you speed up the more fluency you experience?
- Do you slow down before anticipating a stammer?
- Do you speed up immediately after stammering?
- Do you find it hard to pause?
- Are there too few pauses in your speech?
- Are the pauses in your speech too long?

4 *Eye contact*

- Do you look away from people when you stammer?
- Do you stare at people when you stammer?
- Do you find it easy or difficult to look at people when they are talking to you?

5 *Facial expression*

- Do you show too little or too much expression on your face when talking?
- Do you show too little or too much expression on your face when listening to someone talking?

Routledge
Taylor & Francis Group

Continued on Handout **25.3** →

6 *Posture*

- Do you adopt a particular posture when you stammer?

- Do you alter your body position when anticipating stammering or after you have stammered?

Breathing

What do you notice about your breathing when you are speaking?

Tick any of the following that you think may apply to you:

- breathing in too often

- not taking enough time to breathe

- taking in too much air

- breathing in only using the upper part of your chest

- trying to speak as you breathe in

- letting out too much air before you start to speak

- trying to speak when running out of air

- gasping for air

- feeling that you cannot get enough air into your lungs

- feeling tight or tense when you breathe in

- feeling tight or tense when you breathe out

- anything else?

....

....

....

....

....

....

Associated body features

1 *Body movements during speech*

When you speak, do you:

- fidget

- move your arms or legs a lot

- change your posture frequently

- fiddle with your hands or an object such as a pen

- clench your hands

- cover your face, eyes, mouth

- jerk your head

- anything else?

....

....

....

....

2 *Body tension during speech*

When you speak, is there tension or tightness which others may or may not notice:

- all over your body

- in your head (increased pressure)

- in your face

- in your neck and shoulders

- in your stomach and chest

- in your arms and legs

- anywhere else?

....

....

....

....

Routledge
Taylor & Francis Group

6 | Covert identification

Following on from the identification of overt features, this chapter continues the process of identification with the focus on the intrinsic or covert features of stammering. We consider these features to be some of the most significant in terms of maintaining the disorder. If they are not managed in a timely way there are concerns that, even if the overt features are temporarily reduced, these covert features will reappear at some later date and the client may return to clinic seeking further help.

When considering the relationship between overt and covert features, both the client and the clinician need to be aware that there is not a direct correlation. One client may stammer very little overtly but have developed complex covert systems; another may have a mild overt stammer and a correspondingly small covert part. One diagnostic method that gives us clues about the extent of the covert stammering is to ask the individual to read aloud or say a specific set of words (such as a name and address) and thereby reveal how much of the stammer is being hidden through avoidance behaviours.

Sheehan's (1958) analogy of the stammering iceberg has proved useful in helping clients to understand stammering and the relative contributions made by the overt and covert components (see Handout 26). It is also helpful as a way of describing the process of therapy: the clinician can outline the beginning of therapy as a gradual identification and then 'exposure' of the covert features, allowing all the stammering to be overt. This is then followed by the application of fluency-controlling strategies and subsequent gaining of control over the remaining features of the overt component.

Covert symptoms

Covert symptoms are harder to define than overt features as the list is perhaps more open-ended. It includes the following:

Avoidances. These tend not to be observed directly by others, but there may be outward signs which give clues to an underlying difficulty. For example, a client who has difficulty saying his first name may use a number of switching and filling strategies to avoid starting sentences with it, for example, 'You ask me what my name is, well, it's Trudy', 'My name is Turnbull, Jackie Turnbull'.

Emotional responses before, during and after stammering. Much has been written about these aspects of covert stammering. Van Riper (1982) describes fear as the most common, especially the expectation of communicative inability, verbal impotence and the momentary loss of self-

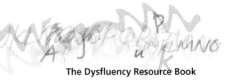

control. He also notes that fear can also be associated with negative listener reactions, social penalties, situations, time pressure, words carrying increased meaning or emotion and specific phonemes or words. More recently, Corcoran & Stewart (1998) have discussed the emotional experiences of adults who stammer. They found suffering was the primary theme of the adults' narratives, with helplessness, shame, fear and avoidance being the four key elements of the suffering.

Clinicians need to be aware of other issues that may arise within the context of discussing covert features of stammering. It is not possible to list all the possibilities here, but some to consider are:

- beliefs about self, such as feelings of inferiority, poor self-esteem and confidence

- perceptions of others, for example, that they attend to stammering more than to the content of the message, that they make judgements about the speaker because of the stammering

- passive or aggressive behaviour, for example, failing to confront difficulties, overreacting to less significant problems

- ways of thinking, such as predicting how things will be in a certain situation before the event has taken place.

Activities to identify covert features

The iceberg ⓘ ⚙

Sheehan's analogy of the iceberg is explained and each client is encouraged to identify relevant personal covert aspects. The 'icebergs' on Handouts 26 and 27 can be used to assist the client in completing this task. It is helpful to look at features experienced:

- before stammering (such as fear, a sense of inevitability or a desire to escape)

- during stammering (such as panic, frustration or embarrassment)

- after stammering (such as relief, anger or shame).

Of course, any of these covert aspects can be experienced at any stage, but looking at stammering in this way ensures that the full range of possible reactions is identified.

An alternative approach is to have clients list the emotional components of their stammering on one iceberg or on three separate ones, using the before, during and after scenario as above. Both a group iceberg (an amalgamation of the feelings and avoidances of the whole group) and individual icebergs (pertinent to each client) can be drawn. An individual iceberg is particularly useful as it often forms the basis for a stammering manual (see Chapter 7 'Desensitisation').

Home-based activity Checklist of covert features

Handout 28 'Identifying your hidden emotions about stammering' can be used as a home-based exercise which is then brought for discussion in a therapy session. This type of checklist has sometimes provided a client with a vehicle for discussing pertinent issues from his past. Spending time on such topics can be fruitful and a way for the client to let go of some of the emotional baggage of his covert stammering.

Alternatively, the checklist can be used as the basis of discussion in individual or group therapy. Clients get a great deal of support when they begin to realise that their difficult emotions are shared by others. Discussing individual checklists in a group or in pairs is therefore cathartic and 'normalising'.

Topic-based discussions

Rather than talk about their emotions directly, some clients respond more readily to topic-based conversations. The emotional component of stammering can be brought to the surface by addressing some of the perceived historical bases of a client's difficulties. For example, when talking about school a client may recall situations in which he was teased or bullied and this may provide an opportunity to discuss any anger he might feel about his stammer.

Home-based activity *Preparation for discussion*
The client is provided with a list of topics (see Handout 29 'Exploring the hidden part of your stammer') from which he chooses three or four which he thinks are pertinent to his stammer. He then writes a short summary of the key points and this is used as a starting point for a discussion with the clinician.

Reflecting on situations

Home-based activity *Anticipating stammering*
The client is asked to consider a number of situations in which he anticipates stammering (see Handout 30 'Important situations') and write down all the feelings he has:

- before
- during
- after stammering.

The emotions identified in this exercise and others in this section form the basis for both identification discussions and therapeutic work described in Chapter 7 'Desensitisation'.

Role plays

Activity role plays can be useful in helping clients to work out what they actually feel and do in relation to the stammer. Two examples are described here.

Telling someone about stammering ⓘ ⚙
Working with a partner, a client role plays telling them about the covert aspects of his stammer, and the partner (or the clinician) asks for detailed clarification. This can also be desensitising and as such is a useful preparation for when a client actually does tell people about stammering. (Students can also be used as listeners for this task; this has the added advantage of helping future clinicians gain greater understanding of the covert nature of stammering from a client perspective rather than from a textbook.)

Discussion *Consideration of possible outcomes* ⓘ ⚙
The previous task can lead to a discussion about what the client predicts will happen when he does the task 'for real'. The client should be encouraged to consider the following:

- the worst case scenario
- the best case scenario
- at least three other possible outcomes.

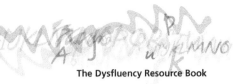

The client and/or the group then problem solve strategies for dealing with such eventualities. In reality, the worst thing rarely, if ever, happens. However, if the client feels he knows what to do should it occur, he is more willing to try telling someone about his stammer. By considering a range of possibilities the client begins to realise that there are a number of ways in which people might respond – and that many or most of them are likely to be positive.

Predicting a situation ⚙

One client describes a stammering situation and predicts how it might happen, were it to occur at some point in the next few days. He predicts how he might feel and think, and how he might stammer. He predicts how the others in the situation might appear and how they might respond to his stammering.

The situation is then role played with other group members acting as other people in the scenario. (If time permits the scene may be replayed again with group members taking other roles.)

A discussion then takes place comparing the predictions the client made with his experiences in the role play and those of the other group members. It sometimes happens, of course, that the person's predictions are validated. If this is the case it is important to look at why it has occurred. Strategies for dealing with a similar situation need to be discussed. If the group members react differently from the client's predictions, then that too forms the basis for discussion alongside the 'fluent' clinician's perspective.

Another lesson that can be learned from this kind of experience is that predicting situations in such a 'tight' or rigid way actually does not help. It is better to experiment with a more open approach alongside desensitising techniques and to encourage the aim of good communication, regardless of the level of stammering.

Other activities for identifying covert stammering

Exploring covert stammering through a visual image ⓘ ⚙

A client is asked to represent his stammer visually. It is important to emphasise that expert drawing or artistic abilities are not required; rather it is an alternative method of communication, another way of explaining how the stammer is for the client. There should be a variety of mediums available (for example chalk, charcoal, wax, pencils, felt tips, coloured and plain paper, collage materials). The client should be encouraged to make a representation, with the clinician observing and discussing the feelings evoked while the work is taking place.

Different clients approach this task in different ways. Some focus mainly on overt features, but the majority portray a sense of what it feels like to stammer. We are often presented with images of 'hurdles' to get over or 'burdens' to be born. Walls and confined spaces with little or no obvious escape route frequently figure as examples of the former. The latter are often illustrated using images such as shackles or heavy weights. These representations give an enormous scope for discussion.

The following are questions to ask while the image is being constructed:

• Why have you chosen that paper/colour/image?

• How do the parts of the image relate to one another: why are those two things together, why is there a space there?

• What are your feelings as you make this image?

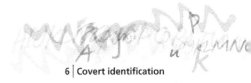
- What are your thoughts as you make this image?

These are questions to ask once the image is finished:

- How do you feel now that you have finished?

- In what way does it represent the hidden part of your stammer?

- Has it always felt like this, or when has it felt different, and how?

- If you were to make another image, of 'your ideal' speech, how would that be different?

- What would have to happen to make this image more like your ideal?

It is important to discuss with the client what he wishes to do with the image that has been created; that is, if it is to be kept, who will keep it and where. If it is to be destroyed, who will destroy it, and how?

Images can be used to track a client's progress through therapy and record a final outcome. (For further discussion of this see Stewart & Brosh, 1997.)

Discussion The advantages and disadvantages of stammering and of fluency ⚙

Clients discuss the advantages and disadvantages of stammering and then of fluency. We include both titles as this can encourage clients to consider the issues in a more open way. It can be useful to have clients take opposing sides in a debate rather than have clinicians defending, for example, the disadvantages of fluency. This can be a useful identification exercise, as many feelings are brought into the open for discussion.

If your clients struggle to come up with advantages of stammering, then here are a few that clients have mentioned to us in the past. Stammering:

- increases your sensitivity to others

- makes you more aware of other people's vulnerability

- makes you more caring

- makes you more tolerant

- makes you more patient.

Activity for consolidating identification work

'Stammer like me manual' ⓘ ⚙

Using the completed checklists on identification (the overt, covert and avoidance features on Handouts 25, 28 and 31), a client is asked to compile an 'instruction manual' for his stammer, the 'Stammer like me manual'. He reads it first to the clinician and then to the group, who ask him questions about it. Some clients will need to build up to the group presentation by, for example, reading their manual first to a significant other, then to one group member, then to a small subgroup, and so on.

Avoidance

While we include a separate chapter on avoidance reduction (Chapter 9), the issue of identifying avoidances requires some additional explanation here. We have incorporated the identification of avoidance behaviours in the identification process for the following reasons:

- It is frequently a huge issue for many, if not most, of our clients.
- It can be difficult for clients to identify avoidances as they occur continually, often at a subconscious or automatic level.
- It can be difficult for clients to work on.

By identifying and then reducing avoidances, the person learns to accept and cope more effectively with his stammer and thus maximise his communication potential.

Types of avoidance

Sheehan's five levels (1975) remain a very useful way of looking at avoidance. Clients may be aware of some of their avoidances at some of the levels, but often they are not aware of the extent of their avoidances at other levels. (A more detailed description of the five levels is given in Chapter 9. A brief summary is included here for clarity.)

Word avoidance: this refers to the myriad ways in which someone will avoid saying a word on which he perceives he will stammer (for example, substituting a word, altering word order).

Situation avoidance: the specific situations or groups of situations a person does not engage in (for example, using the phone, speaking in groups).

Feeling avoidance: expressing an emotion which the person believes will disrupt his fluency or a general approach to expressing feelings (for example, becoming angry, being open about his feelings to another person).

Relationship avoidance: making relationships, for example, with the opposite sex. Restrictions may be imposed on some relationships because stammering is construed as a taboo subject which neither the speaker nor the listener feels they can mention.

Ego protective/self role avoidance: the avoidance of accepting self as a person who stammers, meaning that the person does not live harmoniously with his stammer and does all he can to hide it from others.

Activities to identify avoidance behaviour

Avoidance checklist ❶ ⚙

Using Handout 31 'Avoidance checklist', which describes the different types of avoidance, clients read a section at a time and then explain what they understand of what they have read to the clinician and/or other group members, outlining how it applies to them.

Discussion topics ❶ ⚙

Using the headings on Handout 31, a client or group of clients chooses to discuss one topic from each level. Discussion of all five levels should be achieved over a number of sessions.

Discussion topics for the five levels of avoidance

Here are some suggestions for discussions the clinician might have with a client or group of clients. The topics are divided into Sheehan's five levels of avoidance, so clinicians can choose to cover all levels or those most relevant to their clients.

Word avoidance

What happens when I try to use words I fear?

Why is it that words beginning with ' … ' are so difficult for me to say? (Each client will need to fill in this sentence with the sound relevant for them.)

Is the problem in my speech muscles or in my head?

Does practising the words over and over help my word avoidance?

Situation avoidance

What do I feel when I am in the situation I fear?

Is situation avoidance a problem of anxiety?

It is easier just to live my life skirting round my feared situations.

Am I more concerned about what other people think or my own fear in these situations?

Feeling avoidance

What is the link between what I feel and my stammer?

It is better to keep your emotions under control than express them openly.

I have never been a person who says what they feel. (It is also a feature of my family.)

If you tell people what you feel it upsets them.

Relationship avoidance

I do not have an avoidance issue at this level; it's just that I am not a naturally sociable person.

Stammering has made me shy.

My true friends know I have a stammer and make allowances.

I prefer my own company.

Self role

My stammering makes me who I am.

If I didn't stammer I would have chosen a different career path.

I don't need to talk about my stammer: it's there for all to see and hear.

People who stammer are better in jobs that don't require good communication skills.

Home-based activity An avoidance diary

A client keeps a diary of one aspect of his avoidance (for example, a word or a situation) during a specified period of time and repeats the activity for other aspects. These observations can be used as the basis for later discussion and are also used for compiling the 'Stammer like me manual'. A follow-on activity is for the client to write similar daily entries on non-avoidance activities, for example, times when he said the word he wanted to or carried out the situation he would previously have avoided.

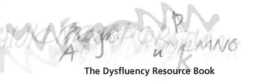
Self-identification

The essential point about self-identification is that the person who stammers sees himself predominantly with respect to the stammer (he is a stammerer and nothing but a stammerer) and fails to fully elaborate other aspects of himself. Dalton (1994) points out that it is all too common for an individual to build a view of self around a problem and to take on the role that society confers on those with that problem. Thus, in self-identification work our aims are threefold:

1   To have the client explore an alternative view(s) of himself.

2   To have the client see his true self and to understand the stammer in the context of that knowledge.

Thorne describes the value of this process as follows:

> Only through as full an understanding as possible of the way in which clients view themselves and the world can the therapist hope to encourage the subtle changes in self concept which make for growth.
> (1990, p117)

3   To reflect back to the client his positive aspects in order to facilitate change.

> … the best clinicians, the most effective clinicians embody the practice of unconditional positive regard. They use themselves as a mirror to reflect back to the client the positive aspects of herself [*sic*] which are most helpful in the change process. 'Look, this is you. Look at what you can do, what potential you have for change.' Looking into the mirror that is me [*sic* the clinician] and seeing this different representation of herself, I hope to enable her to grasp what is possible and gain a new perspective on the self she could be.
> (Stewart, 2005)

Facilitating self-identification

There are a number of ways in which we promote self-identification in the therapy process.

Language of responsibility. Both in individual and group therapy we stress the need for individuals to use the language of responsibility. This is an important way of encouraging a person to see stammering as something he can have some control over, rather than something that happens by itself, in a vacuum. Thus we encourage such phrases as 'I feel nervous/embarrassed/anxious when I stammer' rather than 'my stammer makes me nervous/embarrassed/anxious'. In a group it is also important that people respect each other's individuality and acknowledge that those who stammer are not exactly the same. Thus, members are asked to rephrase such statements as 'People who stammer are worse in interviews' to 'My stammering is worse in interviews' and 'We are introverts' to 'I am an introvert'.

Client-centred therapy. We fully embrace this approach in all therapy we engage in. A client's view is at the centre of their therapy; their priorities become ours.

Creating choice. A client is given choice over the what, when and how of therapy, and any therapeutic targets are negotiated with him.

Target setting outside clinic. Work is directed towards achieving targets outside clinic, in the real surroundings of the client's everyday life.

Significant others and support networks. A client is actively encouraged to involve important others in the therapy process: to have other people attend clinic with him, to help him achieve his targets and basically be a therapist's ally! In addition, we promote the development of support networks, which increase in their significance as the client becomes less dependent on individual and/or group sessions.

We use various psychological approaches as the basis for self-identification work. These have been outlined in the opening chapter. In the following section we will describe a number of activities which have been developed from these approaches, but with relevance to this area.

Activities for self-identification

Problem-free talk ⓘ ⓖ

This idea comes from solution-focused brief therapy (de Shazer, 1985, 1988). In this approach clients are encouraged to look at *solutions* they are using, or could use, rather than exploring the *problem*. They may not be aware of these solutions, for example, solutions that have been used in the past.

One way of exploring these solutions is through problem-free talk. In this procedure a client is invited to talk about any aspect of himself but not about the problem. Clinicians can then feed back positives, for example, 'You seem to be a resourceful/level-headed/caring person', thus helping the client to focus on how he can use his resources to problem solve.
A client is often surprised when a clinician says what he is good at, not what he fails at; it sets a good tone for the relationship. We have found this kind of exploration, with an explanation of its purpose given to the client, to be particularly useful at the beginning of therapy.

Using art and/or visual media ⓘ ⓖ

The section on covert identification discussed how visual images or representations can be used to explore some of the covert aspects of stammering. There are a range of techniques in this area which can be used effectively to help the client gain greater self-understanding. Here are some examples especially pertinent to this client group from Sunderland & Engleheart (1993):

Life graph/life path/the film of your life. In slightly different ways, all of these exercises help a client to explore the significant things that have happened to him over the years and look at how these may be affecting him currently.

Your story. This uses metaphor to help a client gain insight into his life.

Dream time. The aim of this activity is for a client to explore his worst fear(s). It can be adapted to look at fears related to stammering.

You and your jigsaw. This exercise aims to help a client look at his true self and false self, that is, the self he feels is really him and the self he feels he has taken on, for whatever reason.

Gallery of assets. This is an exercise in developing self-esteem by helping a client to think of the things about himself of which he is proud. In a group, the person could be helped to take on board the ideas of other members.

You and your shadow. This is used to help a person become aware of aspects of himself that he is currently denying or hiding and explore why this might be.

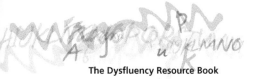

Self-characterisations ⓘ ⚙

These can be seen as a structured way of helping clinicians get in touch with their clients' world. The client maintains the freedom to expose as much or as little as he chooses about that world. Kelly (1991) suggests a specific format to help make such an exercise as unthreatening as possible:

> I want you to write a character sketch of (Harry Brown), just as if he were the principal character in a play. Write it as it might be written by a friend who knew him very intimately and very sympathetically, perhaps better than anyone could ever really know him. Be sure to write it in the third person. For example, start out by saying, '(Harry Brown) is …'
> (1991, p242)

It is important that the client does not see this as a 'test'. We may sometimes need to explain that it does not matter, for example, if he is an untidy writer or a poor speller. If this appears to be a real problem for the client, he can dictate to the clinician. Our aim is to try to understand him as well as we can. Kelly points out that, 'the object of this kind of inquiry is to see how the client structures a world in relation to which he must maintain himself in some kind of role' (1991, p243). Here are some ways we have found which may help you to think about your clients' responses in a one-to-one therapy situation.

- Consider your first reaction to the writing. How does the client come across to you, and what would the world be like as seen through his eyes?
- Pay attention to the first and last sentences of the characterisation. These can be particularly important.
- Is the stammer mentioned? If so, to what extent?
- What possibilities does the client see as being open to him? What restrictions does he place on himself?
- Do any themes run through the writing? If so, what are they?
- Look for cause and effect statements. Kelly points out that these can indicate how the client is likely to approach therapeutic change.
- Is the client specific or general in what he says?
- Are other people, places, situations mentioned, or is the client alone 'in his head'?
- Are the constructs mainly superordinate (more abstract) or subordinate (more behavioural)?
- Does the person use constructs that are tight (those leading to unvarying predictions) or loose (those leading to varying predictions)?
- Are contradictions apparent? If so, are these overtly or covertly expressed? What is the client telling you?
- Look for any constructs that show how clients have approached change in the past. What solutions are mentioned? Are there indications as to the client's attitude to change? Is there a feeling of hope or resignation about problems?
- Is there anything that seems to be missing?

Self-characterisations can be approached in numerous ways, according to the needs of the particular client. These are just some examples of how they can be used:

- as the client is now
- as he was in the past (six months/one year/ten years ago, as appropriate)
- as he would like to be

- as a fluent person

- as a confident person

- as an assertive person

- as he would settle for

- saying the things he wants to (not avoiding)

- being open about his stammer

- feeling in control.

Dalton suggests asking the client to write about himself in terms of 'Who am I apart from my stutter?' (1994, p62). This could also take the form of a self-characterisation.

Self-characterisations can also be written at different times in therapy, enabling clients and clinicians to consider changes that have and have not been made and as a means of assessing the direction for any future therapy.

In a group situation self-characterisations can be used in a number of ways:

- Each person reads his characterisation to the group. The person both 'owns' the things he says and shares important information about himself, often to an extent that he has never done before. Group members then ask questions and make comments. Hayhow & Levy (1989) suggest that questions and answers maintain the third party stance to give some distance and protection. Someone might ask, for example, 'What does this person wish he could tell his wife about his stammer?', to which the reply might be, 'He would like to tell her just how inferior it makes him feel'.

- Group members can suggest appropriate titles for other members' self-characterisations.

- Specific constructs may be chosen for 'laddering' or 'pyramiding' in front of the group. (For further information on these procedures see Button, 1985; Dalton & Dunnett, 1989; Hayhow & Levy, 1989; Jackson, 1989.)

Noticing unhelpful thinking ⓘ ⚙

Many people who stammer (and many who don't!) have distorted and unhelpful thinking patterns of which they are often unaware. Helping clients to notice their own unhelpful ways of thinking can be illuminating and is the first stage in starting to change them. We use Handout 32 'Noticing your unhelpful thinking' as a basis for helping clients in this identification process

An example of a stammering iceberg

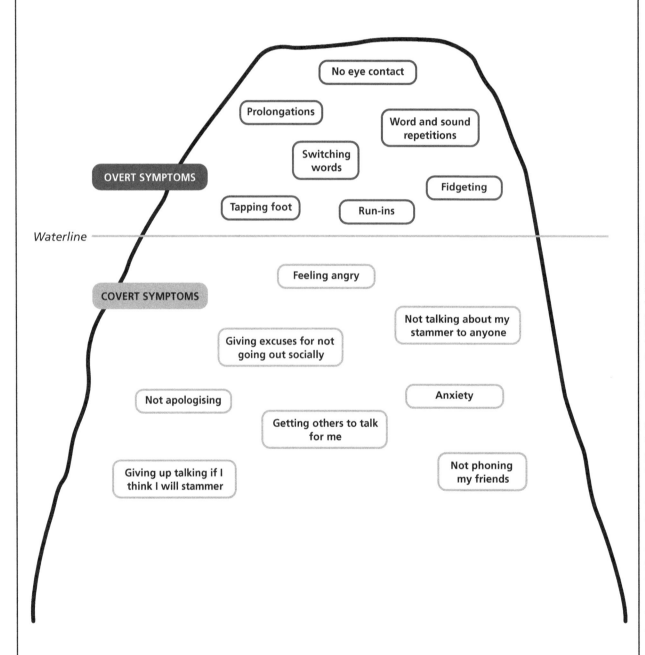

OVERT SYMPTOMS

No eye contact

Prolongations

Word and sound repetitions

Switching words

Fidgeting

Tapping foot

Run-ins

Waterline

COVERT SYMPTOMS

Feeling angry

Not talking about my stammer to anyone

Giving excuses for not going out socially

Not apologising

Anxiety

Getting others to talk for me

Giving up talking if I think I will stammer

Not phoning my friends

Routledge
Taylor & Francis Group

The iceberg (blank)

OVERT SYMPTOMS

Waterline

COVERT SYMPTOMS

Routledge
Taylor & Francis Group

Identifying your hidden emotions about stammering

Think about the feelings you experience associated with your stammering. Identifying them can be quite painful because it brings you face to face with some very difficult emotions. However, you need to be sure about what it is you are actually feeling and why you feel the way you do if you are to make any changes.

Here are some emotions people who stammer say they feel. Some will be familiar to you, others may not. Consider which ones are relevant to you, and why.

Embarrassment

Do you feel embarrassed when you stammer? If so, why is this? Here are a few possibilities. Do these apply to you, or are there other reasons why you feel embarrassed?

- You think other people will be embarrassed by your speaking and you react accordingly.
- You do not say the things you really mean or want to say but instead say what you can say fluently.
- You feel your speech lets you down and makes people think less well of you.
- You feel inferior to others because you stammer.
- Other reasons:

....

....

....

....

Anxiety/fear

Do you feel anxious about stammering? If so, is this worse before you talk to someone or while you are talking to them? Are any of the following reasons for anxiety relevant to you?

- You fear being judged negatively because of your stammer.
- You feel you need to be constantly 'on guard', scanning ahead for difficult words, and are therefore unable to relax in the conversation.
- You spend a great deal of time trying not to stammer and being afraid that your listener will find out.
- Other reasons:

....

....

....

....

....

Shame

Often people tell us they feel ashamed of their stammering. If this is true for you, ask yourself the following questions:

- Do you feel others think your stammer makes you inferior in some way?
- Do you think people feel sorry for you?
- Do you feel different?
- Do you feel you should be able to talk like everyone else and somehow it is your fault if you do not?

This page may be photocopied for instructional use only. The Dysfluency Resource Book © J Turnbull & T Stewart 2010

Continued on Handout 28.2 →

• Other reasons:

....

....

....

....

....

Anger

Anger is often associated with stammering. Sometimes the anger is directed at yourself, sometimes at other people. Are you angry with any of the following?

• Yourself for not being able to control your speech.

• Your parents for not reacting appropriately to you when you were younger, not talking to you about the stammer or not taking you to therapy.

• Other people for not being patient, or for laughing or finishing your words, and so on.

• Other people for being fluent when talking can be so effortful for you.

• Other people or reasons:

....

....

....

....

....

Sadness

Do you feel a sense of sadness about your speech? Does stammering frequently make you feel unhappy? Do you think about it a lot of the time? Which of the following cause sadness?

• You feel different.

• You feel you have missed out on things in the past and cannot regain them.

• You have not done the things you wanted to with your life; you have let the stammer decide what you can and cannot do.

• You envisage a future of missed opportunities.

• Other reasons:

....

....

....

....

....

Routledge
Taylor & Francis Group

H28.2

Exploring the hidden part of your stammer

Choose topics from the list below that you think are significant in exploring the hidden part of your stammer. Write a short summary of the key points under each topic, ready to discuss with your clinician.

Family life

....

....

....

School times

....

....

....

Coping with stammering as a child

....

....

....

Being an adolescent

....

....

Making friends and developing relationships

....

....

....

Making decisions, eg subject choices at school, career path, choosing a job, applying for university

....

....

....

....

Important relationships in my life

....

....

....

Self-belief and keeping my confidence

....

....

....

Positive memories/sparkling moments

....

....

....

Routledge
Taylor & Francis Group

Important situations

Write down the feelings you experience in these situations.

The telephone

....

....

....

Queuing

....

....

....

Talking to people in authority

....

....

....

Talking in groups

....

....

....

Presentations

....

....

....

Banter and small talk

....

....

....

Going out (eg pub, restaurant, cinema, theatre, socialising)

....

....

....

Interviews

....

....

....

Formal situations (eg weddings)

....

....

....

Asking for something

....

....

....

Answering questions

....

....

....

Shopping

....

....

....

Dealing with difficult listeners

....

....

....

Talking to family members

....

....

....

Routledge
Taylor & Francis Group

Avoidance checklist

Joseph Sheehan wrote about five levels of avoidance*. Each level is listed below. Consider each one in turn and think about how it relates to you and your stammering.

Word avoidance

Are you aware of avoiding particular words?

Make a list of words you know you avoid saying.

....

....

Do you:

- sometimes avoid saying particular words altogether, eg by omitting them or switching them for an alternative?

- pretend you have forgotten a word?

- pretend not to have heard so you do not have to reply?

- do something else as you say the word, to create a distraction, eg cough, drop something, change position?

- change the order of words?

- add extra words in order to 'put off' saying the difficult word?

- have 'run-ins' into what you are saying, eg 'What I mean to say is …'?

- give up speaking altogether on occasions?

- put on accents or funny voices, or pretend to be angry to get yourself over a difficult word?

If so, what is it about the words that make them difficult to say? Is it:

- the sound they start with?

- the length of the word?

- the meaning they convey?

- the circumstance in which the word is said?

What do you feel would happen if you went ahead and said the word? Have you tried in the past? If so, what happened?

....

....

Situation avoidance

Are there situations you avoid because you fear stammering? Make a list of what they are.

....

....

....

How often do you avoid them? Do you avoid because of:

- particular sorts of people?

- the number of people present?

- the activity involved, such as using the phone, having to give your name?

- the type of situation, such as a party, a crowded pub, a queue, a busy shop?

- what you would have to say?

- what you fear others might say, do or think if they heard you stammer?

What do you fear would happen if you did enter the situation?

....

....

....

* Sheehan JG (1975) 'Conflict theory and avoidance reduction therapy', Eisenson J (ed), *Stuttering: A Second Symposium,* Harper & Row, New York.

Continued on Handout **31.2** →

Routledge

What has happened before?

....

....

....

Feeling avoidance

Do you avoid expressing particular emotions and/or find some feelings hard to express? Make a list of what they are.

....

....

How often would you say you avoid expressing them?

Why do you think you avoid them?

....

....

....

Are they connected with:

- saying something positive, such as giving praise, saying thank you?

- requesting help, asking a favour?

- saying something negative, such as criticising, expressing anger?

- saying how you feel at a particular moment: sad, expressing concern or affection?

- apologising?

Why do you think these emotions are hard for you to express?

....

....

....

What do you fear would happen if you stammered while expressing them?

....

....

....

Relationship avoidance

Are there any relationships that you think are affected by your stammering? Make a list of any that concern you.

....

....

....

Are there times when you feel unable to form friendships because you are concerned about your stammering?

....

....

....

How does your stammer affect your current friendships?

....

....

....

....

This page may be photocopied for instructional use only. *The Dysfluency Resource Book* © J Turnbull & ⁻ Stewart 2010

Routledge
Taylor & Francis Group
ROUTLEDGE

Continued on Handout **31.3** →

H31.₂

Do you feel you are less open in relationships because you stammer?

....

....

....

Do you feel less confident about yourself in relationships because of your stammer?

....

....

....

Self role avoidance

Sheehan (1975, p157) said, 'Stuttering is a false-role disorder. You will remain a stutterer so long as you pretend not to be one'.
List the ways you think you try to avoid being a person who stammers.

....

....

....

How open are you about your stammer: do you mention it to others? If so, how freely? If not, why not?

....

....

....

Do you ever 'comment' on your stammer, for example by saying, 'I'm having a bad day' or 'That was a hard word for me to say'?

....

....

....

Is it more important to you to say the things you want to and risk stammering or to say something different but fluently?

....

....

....

Do you accept your stammer or do you try to hide it as much as possible?

....

....

....

What would be the consequences of being open and allowing yourself to stammer?

....

....

....

Routledge
Taylor & Francis Group

Noticing your unhelpful thinking

Most of us have times when we look at things in ways which are not helpful to us. Learning to recognise these 'thinking errors' is the first step to considering other, more helpful, ways of thinking. We may not be able to change a situation, but we can consider alternative and more helpful ways of looking at it.

Below are some of the common thinking errors that people may experience. Have a look and ask yourself if any of these are ways in which you typically think. If they are, write down an example from your own experience.

All or nothing thinking

We look at things in an absolute or extreme way and see them as either black or white, with no shades of grey.

Example: If you are on a diet and you eat a chocolate bar, you think you are a failure.

Example: If you stammer in a shop, you believe everyone thinks you are stupid.

An example of your own:

....

....

Over-generalisation

We see one negative event as part of a repetitive pattern or make an overall conclusion from a single event.

Example: You fail to win the lottery and say, 'I never have good luck'.

Example: Someone laughs at you when you stammer and you say to yourself, 'Everyone thinks stammering is funny'.

An example of your own:

....

....

Negative mental filter

We dwell on the negative things that happen and often don't even notice the positives.

Example: Someone points out a spelling mistake in something you have written which they tell you is otherwise excellent and you only think about the mistake, not about any other aspect.

Example: You stammer in an interview and think the whole interview is a disaster.

An example of your own:

....

....

Ignoring the positives

We don't accept that the good things we have done are of any worth. We think they are not good enough or that anyone else could have done just as well. Positive things become negative ones in your mind.

Example: You spend time making a really nice meal, but when complimented say that it could have been much better and it was just thrown together.

Example: You make a complicated phone call, saying all you need to and getting what you want from the conversation, but discount it because you stammer.

An example of your own:

....

....

This page may be photocopied for instructional use only. *The Dysfluency Resource Book* © J Turnbull & T Stewart 2010

Routledge
Taylor & Francis Group

Continued on Handout 32.2 →

Jumping to conclusions

There are two ways in which we do this:

1   Mind reading – we assume things about people without any evidence.

Example: Someone in a crowd doesn't wave at you and you assume they are ignoring you.

2   Fortune telling – we predict things will turn out badly.

Example: You have to meet someone new and you 'know' before you meet them that they will be embarrassed if you stammer.

An example of your own:

....

....

Magnification/minimisation

We either (1) exaggerate things out of all proportion (sometimes called 'catastrophising'), or (2) minimise their importance.

Example: (1) A friend cancels an arrangement at the last minute, saying she feels unwell. You realise you have forgotten her birthday, assume she is upset and does not want to continue the friendship.

Example: (2) You are complimented on the way you explained something but, because you stammered, you see it as insignificant that someone thanked you for making it so clear.

An example of your own:

....

....

Emotional reasoning

Feelings are mistaken for facts: we feel in a particular way and therefore assume this is how we are.

Example: I feel impatient. I am an uncaring person.

Example: I feel anxious. I can't express myself properly.

An example of your own:

....

....

Thinking in extremes

We use words like 'should'/'shouldn't'/'must'/ 'ought' to criticise ourselves and others. This sort of thinking is very rigid and can be hard to change.

Example: Someone asks you to go to a film that you have absolutely no interest in seeing. You tell yourself, 'They should know it's not a film I would enjoy'.

Example: You go for an interview and you tell yourself, 'I mustn't stammer'.

An example of your own:

....

....

Labelling

We give ourselves negative labels when something negative happens rather than just saying we have made a mistake.

Example: You stammer and say, 'I can't put my point across'.

An example of your own:

....

....

This page may be photocopied for instructional use only. *The Dysfluency Resource Book* © J Turnbull & T Stewart 2010

Routledge

Taking all the responsibility and blaming

We take events personally and blame ourselves or others for things we or they are not responsible for.

Example: You break a cup when arguing with your partner and say, 'Look what you've made me do'.

Example: Someone puts the phone down on you when you block and you blame yourself for stammering.

An example of your own:

....

....

Routledge
Taylor & Francis Group

7 | Desensitisation

Desensitisation refers to a change in the emotions a person feels regarding stammering, especially fear. Indeed, Williams simply calls desensitisation 'fear reduction' (1979, p246), while Gregory talks about 'reduction of fear-arousing stimuli including the occurrence of stuttering' (1979, p17). Similarly, Van Riper, who devotes a whole chapter of his book *The Treatment of Stuttering* to this topic, refers to 'calming and toughening the stutterer' (1973, p367) and to 'the ways by which we seek to reduce the stutterer's speech anxieties and other disturbing emotional states' (1973, p267). Levy prefers to construe desensitisation from a personal construct psychology perspective, calling it 'reconstruing stuttering' (1987, p110), and sees its purpose as helping the person 'to stutter openly without experiencing unpleasant reactions' (p111).

Desensitisation has its roots in the work of Bryngelson, Johnson and Van Riper at the University of Iowa in the 1930s. Instead of setting out to give their clients fluency (which they felt would not be maintained), these clinicians developed an approach based on *modifying* the stammer and *reducing the negative emotions* connected with stammering (the 'stammer more fluently' school; Gregory, 1979). Today, desensitisation is seen as an essential and major part of most therapeutic interventions and as crucial to the maintenance of change.

Van Riper (1973) outlines three targets of desensitisation: (1) the confrontation of the disorder, (2) the core behaviour, described as raising the client's tolerance 'for fixations and oscillations' (Van Riper, 1973, p274), and (3) resisting communicative stress and listener penalty.

When to use

Work on desensitisation is likely to be a fundamental aspect of therapy with most clients, although for a few this is not the case. In our clinical practice we occasionally come across those for whom the covert part of the stammer is very small; they may or may not also have a small overt component to the stammer. Such people find the stammer little more than an inconvenience or a frustration and can benefit considerably from therapy directed almost exclusively towards behaviour change. Some may only present for therapy when confronted by a particular life event (such as having to make a speech) for which they are seeking specific techniques. It is, however, important that this area is fully investigated during the identification stage, as some people discover after such exploration that they are in fact not as desensitised as they originally thought.

Desensitisation aims to change the way stammering is construed and to help the person learn to view it as something he does, rather than as something he is. A person who stammers often

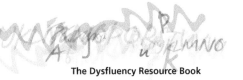

has little choice as to whether or not he stammers. He can, however, develop choices about both *how* he stammers and how he *feels* about stammering. Desensitisation is the process by which such feelings can be modified. It should start very early in therapy and, indeed, much of the work in identification also involves an element of desensitisation as the client confronts head on something he has been trying to hide or deny for so long. As Manning points out, 'it is difficult to critically identify and analyse one's behaviour and attitudes without achieving at least some distance and objectivity' (2000, p282). When using a solution-focused perspective, work on desensitisation follows smoothly on from identification of a preferred future in which stammering is no longer as problematic for the client.

Desensitisation will frequently be worked on in parallel with avoidance reduction. Changing thoughts about and attitudes towards stammering will be most productive when there is a concurrent change in behaviour. Sometimes the behaviour change comes first and produces the attitude change; at other times it is a change in attitude which can allow a behaviour change to take place. Which comes first may vary according to the individual and sometimes the same person will benefit from both types of approach at different times. For example, a person may fear introducing himself and therefore always wait to be introduced. He may work first on the behaviour, taking the plunge and introducing himself. He may learn from this experience that, although he stammers, if he uses good eye contact the other person will respond positively. This can lead to a reduction of anticipatory fear the next time such a situation arises. On the other hand, he may prefer to examine his fears first before he carries out the behaviour. The clinician can use Socratic questioning (see Chapter 1, the section 'CBT and stammering therapy', p10) to help the client examine the validity of his thoughts, and only when he has done so will he feel able to alter his behaviour.

Teaching desensitisation

There are many ways in which desensitisation can be approached in therapy. Before specific 'exercises' are carried out, however, it is important that the rationale for this kind of work is fully explained and is agreed and accepted by clients (see Handout 33). It is very hard for some people to confront their stammering and give up old ways of self-protection. Without an understanding of this and agreement that such change is necessary, it is likely that the old ways of coping will feel too entrenched to be resisted. The clinician should be aware that for some clients desensitisation will take a long time. Group therapy can be very helpful in this process, especially an open group where clients are at different stages and 'older' members can share their own experiences of the value of working in this way.

Work on desensitisation starts for many clients before they reach the speech and language therapy clinic. Some will have told significant people in their lives about this step they are taking in seeking help. Others will have read information from self-help organisations or other literature, most of which will probably have at least alluded to the emotional aspects of stammering. Anything a client has done towards his own desensitisation should be reinforced by the clinician, as it demonstrates important changes the person has attempted to make without professional help. Desensitisation continues in therapy in the identification phase, in specific activities listed below, but also in ongoing discussion with the clinician, group members and other people in the client's life.

NB It is extremely important that a client is aware that in becoming desensitised to stammering, his overt stammer may become worse for a time. This is because he is facing head on the feelings and behaviours he may have tried very hard to hide. Most clients come

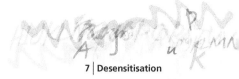

to therapy expecting as least some increase in fluency. Finding that his stammering increases initially can be very distressing if the client has not been warned of this possibility and the reason for it.

Common problems

- The client finds it too threatening to work on desensitisation because he is still at a stage of contemplation (Prochaska & DiClemente, 1992). He needs further time to consider the implications of change.

- The client has come to therapy for fluency. He wants to change his speech, not his feelings.

- The client fears the accompanying increase in dysfluency that he has been told may accompany this process.

- The client does not have the support of his family, friends and/or work associates, who may want him to continue hiding his stammer for reasons of their own.

Principles of desensitisation

Do not rush work on desensitisation. At the same time, it is also important to be aware that sometimes a client, once he realises the importance of this work, can become desensitised far more quickly that the clinician might expect. We must always remember to work at a pace appropriate to the client. Generally, it is best to work in small, achievable steps and build on previous successes.

It is usually easier for a person to start working on desensitisation with people and in surroundings where he feels safest. However, the clinician should not assume that she knows with whom or where this might be. For example, one person may find it easier to talk to family members about stammering, while another may find a stranger less threatening.

Tolerating silence/time pressure

For many who stammer, silence is associated with not being able to speak. Thus, a person often feels a need to continue speaking without pausing and there seems to be a sense of urgency, even compulsion, about his communication. Urgency about communication can result in an 'I've started so I'll finish' sort of approach to speaking. Speech is not only rushed but contains few pauses and as a consequence the listener may find it hard to take in what is being said. Listener reactions can then be misinterpreted by the person who stammers as negative reactions to the stammer itself.

Activities for increasing tolerance of silence/time pressure

Ceasing to talk at a signal ⓘ ⚙
With the clinician or another group member, a client talks on a given or chosen topic.

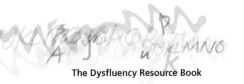
At a non-verbal signal from his partner or the clinician, he has to cease talking until given a signal to recommence. The length of the silence can be increased as the speaker's tolerance increases, as can the amount of eye contact required from him. Listeners may also try to encourage the speaker to give way to time pressure, while the speaker aims to remain calm in the face of such pressure. Feelings aroused by this experience are then shared. Ensuing discussion may include exploration of situations in which people experience such pressure and experiments for practice can be set up both in the clinical situation and outside.

Holding eye contact ⓘ ⚙

With the clinician or another group member, a client talks on a given or self-chosen topic. When it is his turn to speak, he has to hold eye contact with the listener and remain silent for a specified amount of time before starting to speak again.

Speaking circles ⚙

Speaking circles were described by Lee Glickstein (1989), not for people who stammer, but to help people in general who wanted to develop their communication skills and reduce their fear of group and public speaking. It was Harrison (2000) who developed the use of these circles with people who stammer. One of the main aims of speaking circles is desensitisation. The procedure we use is described below.

Group members and the clinician sit in a semicircle. Each person in turn stands in front of the group and connects with their audience for at least 30 seconds by making soft eye contact (not staring) with all members. (We usually ask for a volunteer to start and then to choose the next speaker, and so on.)

After the time has elapsed the clinician signals to the speaker, who can then either elect to remain silent, continuing to make eye contact, or speak for the remaining period of time that has been agreed, or do a combination of the two. He can speak on any subject he chooses. We usually set the time for this part of the activity at between one and two minutes depending on the size of the group and the time available for the activity as a whole.

The clinician signals the time is over by starting to clap and is joined in this by the other group members.

The speaker remains standing while two or three group members give brief positive feedback. The feedback is less about content and more about delivery. It is about how the speaker personally impacted on the listener.

The speaker receives the feedback but does not comment on it.

Once all group members have had their turn there is a second round where the 'speaking' section is a little longer.

Although a client may find this a difficult task initially, he will find the absence of judgement and the positive feedback very affirming. The process can be a useful tool in helping a person to see himself in a less negative light and to acknowledge his positive qualities. Stammering no longer feels so risky in such an accepting atmosphere. The more people participate in speaking circles, the less anxious they tend to feel (and this goes for the clinicians too!).

Home-based activity Pausing

Activities for pausing found in Chapter 12 'Rate control' can also be used for desensitisation.

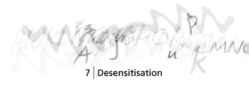

Tolerating stammering

Van Riper (1986) advocates building a client's tolerance to his frustration about communication as a prerequisite to and preparation for modifying the actual behaviour. He proposes that if the person can begin to tolerate his blocks, he is reacting in a new way which will serve him in good stead for further modification work.

Activities for increasing tolerance of stammering

The first two activities are suggested by Van Riper (1973) as ways of building tolerance to frustration.

Freezing ⓘ ⚙

In pairs or with the clinician, at a signal from his partner the client continues the moment of stammering (for example, he freezes his articulators or continues to repeat a sound or word) for an increased length of time. (This is also described in activities in Chapter 14 'Block modification', where this exercise is also appropriate for slightly different reasons.)

'The stammering bath' ⓘ ⚙

This is suggested as an activity for an individual who has a substantial covert component to his stammer. The client sets out to 'collect' a specified (large) number of stammers by allowing himself to stammer overtly rather than hiding his stammer. Such an activity can help in increasing the approach to stammering and decreasing the avoidance components of stammering. This is clearly likely to be a difficult task for many and may need to be worked on using a hierarchy. The person may start by stammering more in the clinic, then with someone he feels at ease with, building up to doing it in increasingly difficult situations.

'Advertising' stammering

Many clients regard their stammering so negatively that they feel they must hide it at all cost. A person may believe that others will construe it in the same way and that if he talks about it to them he will be judged in a poor light. Helping him to test this hypothesis can be illuminating. We feel the concept of 'advertising' stammering has a positive ring to it, with stammering seen as something to be talked about rather than something to be explained, hidden away or apologised for.

Activities to encourage talking about stammering

Talking about emotions aroused by stammering ⓘ ⚙

With the clinician, in pairs or in the whole group, clients talk about past and present examples of stammering and are encouraged to be aware of the emotions aroused as they do so. Exploring feelings in a relatively safe environment is a very useful precursor to doing the same in the 'real' world. However, it is important not to assume that talking about stammering with speech and language clinicians and others who stammer will be easy. Letting out previously well-controlled emotions can be very painful, regardless of the audience. Subjects that we have found to be fertile areas for discussion include the following:

- childhood memories
- problems in relationships
- parental attitudes to stammering
- school experiences with peers and teachers
- advice given in the past
- adverse listener reactions
- unrealised aspirations.

Survey 🎲

Group members are asked to carry out a survey on stammering with members of the public. Reactions tend to start with horror and disbelief, and extend to terror and refusal to participate! Despite this, both we and our clients have found this activity to be one of the most helpful of all the desensitisation exercises. After reassurances that no one will be coerced into participating and that those who do not wish to conduct a survey can just be observers, we go on to describe what will happen. We suggest that clients work in pairs; perhaps a pair will involve someone who is more enthusiastic about the activity working with someone who is less so. Individual clients then think up questions to which they would be personally interested in finding answers. These vary a great deal but tend to include the following areas:

Personal knowledge about stammering. Do you have any friends or relatives who stammer? Have you ever met anyone who stammers? Do you know what stammering is?

Ideas about causation. What do you think causes stammering? Is stammering a medical, psychological or some other sort of problem? What sort of people stammer?

Ideas about treatment. What do you think can be done about stammering? What treatment is available? Have you heard of speech and language therapy?

Feelings about stammering. How do you feel when you talk to someone who stammers? Do you find it easy to talk to someone who stammers? What do you find difficult about talking to someone who stammers?

Reactions to people who stammer. What do you do when speaking to someone who stammers? What do you think is the most helpful way of reacting?

Having sorted out about four or five questions for each pair to ask, the group looks at ways of approaching people, asking questions, dealing with refusals and difficult responses and closing the interview. They practise this in role play, together with any techniques they wish to employ (such as voluntary stammering, block modification, rate control and good eye contact). Each pair decides how many people they will ask and what sort of mix they would like to include (young/old, male/female, leisurely/in a hurry), and so on. Venues for each group are determined, with each pair going to a different place. Clipboards and identity badges can help clients 'look the part' and boost their confidence in approaching the task. Ideas are discussed as to how results will be collated and feedback presented. Then comes the moment of truth – the pairs go off to do the surveys while the clinicians get the kettle on in preparation for their return!

When group members return, we find that the majority are usually positive about the experience. In fact, some are quite exhilarated. Frequently, those who set off only to be observers have decided to have a go, having first seen their partner in action. We allow adequate time for clients to talk about their experiences and then the group members are given the task of making some sort of presentation to the group at the next meeting. This usually contains elements of some or all of the following: (1) a factual report on replies received; (2) feedback on their own and/or their partner's general performance, and on speech and communication, including any skills which were targeted for practice; (3) comments on emotions experienced; and (4) a summary on the usefulness of the survey and what was learned through it.

Interestingly, despite high levels of initial resistance, we have found that some clients decide to repeat this activity on their own as they have found it so beneficial.

Home-based activity 1

The client is asked to make a hierarchy from the easiest to the most difficult people to tell about his stammering and/or speech and language therapy (a sample hierarchy is given in Chapter 15 'Maintenance: a continuing process of change'). He begins by telling the easiest person and works up. He may discover a whole variety of responses. These tend to be mostly positive (people are genuinely interested, concerned to help or surprised to discover that the person has any difficulty in speaking). Sometimes the responses are indifferent (the person is uninterested, takes the conversation no further or changes the subject). Occasionally, there is indeed a negative reaction (embarrassment or amusement or hostility). It is important that the clinician does not try to reassure the client when he reports negative responses, but discusses them objectively.

Discussion ⓘ ⚙

The information received becomes fruitful ground for discussion of questions such as:

- How did you broach the subject?

- What did you say?

- How did you say it (assertively or apologetically)?

- What response did you anticipate?

- What response did you get?

- How did you follow up the response?

- What did the experience teach you?

In a group setting clients gain the advantage of hearing the experiences of others, offering and receiving alternative explanations for some responses and giving suggestions for future approaches to talking about stammering.

Home-based activity 2

The client uses the hierarchy from Home-based activity 1 (or a new one if it is more appropriate) to talk about his stammer (overt and/or covert) as it occurs or when it is anticipated. For example, after stammering he might say: 'That was a difficult word', 'I always seem to stammer on that word', '"s" is usually a difficult sound for me to say'; when anticipating stammering: 'I might find this word hard to say because I stammer'; having avoided a word: 'I meant to say "xxxx" but it's hard because I often stammer on it so I tend to use another word I can say more easily'.

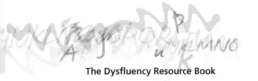
Tolerating difficult listener reactions

It is undoubtedly true that some people react negatively to stammering for a variety of reasons. They may be embarrassed, frustrated, impatient or just inconsiderate. We do our clients no favours by pretending that all listeners will be tolerant if clients are more open. We help clients best by exploring their fears, testing out reality through behavioural experiments and helping them develop coping strategies where necessary.

Activities for tolerating difficult listener reactions

Being laughed at or mocked ⓘ ⚙

In pairs or with the clinician, the client carries out a speaking activity such as reading, describing a room or asking and answering questions. The other person laughs at or mocks him in some way when he stammers. The activity continues until any anxiety aroused has subsided. Care must be taken that this exercise is not exaggerated and therefore lacking in realism. Sensitivity must also be used in deciding when a client is ready for such a task. At the end of the exercise there should be feedback to the clinician or group about the feelings that have been stirred up and the way individuals have tried to deal with them. Any memories that have been awakened can be shared. This can be useful in helping the client to understand some of his feelings about reactions that occur in daily life and why particular reactions affect him more than others.

Speaking to difficult listeners ⚙

Volunteers are needed for this exercise. We use students who, through participating, gain some insights into stammering. The exercise requires plenty of space, ideally as many rooms as there are students. Unbeknown to the clients, the students are each assigned specific difficult listener reactions that they are instructed to display in one-to-one conversations with the clients. Reactions we have used include being patronising, hard of hearing, impatient, bored and over-talkative. Clients are told that we have brought some people in with whom they can practise their speaking skills and that they are to engage them in conversation for about five minutes. After each conversation there is time for both the client and the student to reflect on the client's performance; these reflections are used later in the feedback session. The exercise ends when each student has spoken to each client.

At the end of the exercise the feedback session takes place. Clients tell the group which reactions they found easy to deal with and which were more difficult. Students give feedback on how well they feel the clients dealt with their particular situation. Effective and non-effective strategies are discovered. The notes the students have made about each speaker are summarised and given to the clients at the next group session.

The feedback session is also very important for the students, who often feel quite ambivalent about what they have had to do: they know it is helpful but it goes against all they know about being a good listener. It is important for them to debrief before giving their feedback: for example, 'I am Suzanne, a speech and language therapy student. I was not bored by the conversation'.

NB While we would usually give clients a rationale for all our exercises, we make an exception here. The activity only works well when clients do not know what is going to happen and have to produce coping strategies spontaneously.

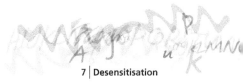

Speaking in difficult situations[1]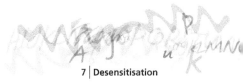

This is a situation role play in which group members are asked to come up with ideas for situations they find problematic. These often include the following:

- asking for a fare on public transport

- returning a faulty item to a shop

- making a complaint to a receptionist

- talking to someone in authority

- explaining something complex in a work situation

- taking part in an interview

- ordering a meal in a restaurant

- asking a shop assistant for an item.

Like the previous activity (speaking to difficult listeners), this exercise involves volunteers and once again we use students. Each of the rooms is set up as a particular scenario (see typical examples in the list above). The students are briefed about the roles they are to play within the scenario and then take up their places in the room and situation.

The task is explained to the group of clients in a central room and a brief description of each scenario is provided for them to read and choose from. A copy of the scenario is fixed to the door of the relevant room to prevent confusion. Each client chooses a scenario and goes to the room. He takes the scenario off the door before entering. (This signifies to other clients wishing to take part in that same role play that it is in use.) The client will replace the scenario details on the door on the way out. After each role play the client returns to the main room and completes a feedback/reflection sheet. He is then free to choose another scenario, or he may repeat the same one.

In the discussion that follows the activity, feedback is given by group members using their reflection sheets, and by volunteers about their observations. Any strategies that might have been useful but were not employed are discussed (see the feedback session in the previous activity).

Nightmare situations

Each group member takes it in turn to outline his worst nightmare (real or imagined) in terms of listener reaction. The group members then role play the situation as it was or as the person fears it would be. After discussion as to what strategies should be used, the situation is replayed using these. Recognising that there can be alternatives is a powerful route to becoming desensitised.

Most disliked reaction

Each group member in turn tells the others the listener reactions he most dislikes. Each person then has a turn to take the chair 'centre stage' and the other group members ask him questions, responding to his answers in the way he dislikes (for example, by laughing or looking away). The group member 'in the chair' responds in ways he feels are most helpful to him (such as ignoring the laughter, challenging the questioner, and so on). At the end of each turn, the effectiveness of the person's reactions to the listeners is discussed.

---

[1] We would like to acknowledge the work of two final year students, Chandy Chima and Samantha Bradley, in developing this activity.

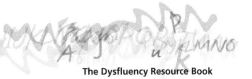

Home-based activity

Bloodstein notes 'the disparity that tends to exist between the listener's attitude and what it is imagined to be' (1975, p73). He suggests helping the client to differentiate between the observation of a behaviour, such as 'he looked away', and the inference of an automatic negative reaction: 'he was embarrassed'. Such work can be incorporated into a home practice task in which the client has to focus on behaviour and is asked to list all possible inferences rather than the one negative one he would have previously come up with. A trusted friend can be asked to help in this task by also observing and then feeding back their (it is to be hoped more objective) findings to the client.

Voluntary stammering

Voluntary stammering is a particularly powerful desensitisation strategy. Because of this it is described and discussed in a chapter of its own (Chapter 8).

Desensitisation

Desensitisation involves changing the way you feel about your stammer and about yourself, too. In this phase of therapy you will learn how to stammer more openly. At the same time you will start to feel differently about stammering as you learn how to deal more effectively with some of the negative feelings you may have, such as shame, embarrassment, anger and fear.

What do I have to do?

During desensitisation you will look at ways to feel calmer when you stammer and toughen yourself to your own and other people's reactions to the stammer. This is not an easy task; you have probably been stammering for many years and your attitudes will not change overnight. It is important that this stage of therapy is not rushed; you need to take small steps so that the changes you make are changes that you can maintain.

There will inevitably be times when you find this process very difficult and you may become disheartened on occasions. It is important that you try to recognise and talk about such feelings with a clinician, a friend or (if you are in a group) with group members. Sharing your frustrations can help you cope better and look at how you can move on.

Activities

Among the activities that are part of desensitisation are the following:

- coping with difficult listener reactions
- coping with silence
- stammering openly and without embarrassment
- tolerating silence
- talking about stammering
- looking at people when you stammer
- voluntary stammering. In this process you stammer in a slow, relaxed and controlled way, and learn that stammering does not have to involve tension and negative feelings.

Routledge
Taylor & Francis Group

8 | Voluntary stammering

Most writers on desensitisation stress the key role that voluntary stammering plays in this process. Some of the proposed additional benefits of voluntary stammering are listed below.

- It helps the person who stammers to be more prepared to take up more of his listeners' time. He is therefore less inclined to impose time pressure on himself (Sheehan, 1975).

- There is a reduction of struggle through the use of repetition in certain situations, specifically those which call for communicative responsibility and the use of propositional language (Eisenson, 1975).

- Johnson saw voluntary stammering as an exercise in throwing caution to the wind by weakening avoidance (Johnson, cited in Bloodstein, 1969).

- It helps the person who stammers to put up with imperfections in fluency, encourages approach not avoidance and allows the person to work on his stammering during fluency, when fear is low (Sheehan, 1986). Sheehan states that the person does not need to know more about fluency; only when he knows how to stutter will he be relaxed and comfortable as a speaker.

- According to Levy (1987), voluntary stammering is particularly useful for interiorised stammerers, as it tackles the fears of stammering directly. It is seen as the opposite of avoidance, which does not permit people to test out their stammering predictions.

While this rationale may make a great deal of sense to clinicians and *logically* be acceptable to clients, clinicians still often need the powers of a superlative salesperson to sell this approach. This is understandable. Mostly clients come to therapy hoping that, even if they will not be 'cured', their fluency will increase. It must feel bewildering, to say the least, when the clinician tells them to do the very thing they want to eradicate and to do it *on purpose!*

One of our clients told us, 'I have not yet made voluntary stammering a lifestyle choice'. It struck us that there was much of interest in what he said. The idea of a 'lifestyle choice' is very apt. Using voluntary stammering is a huge step in the process of coming to terms with stammering and of being able to let go of the sense of shame that may accompany it. By allowing himself to stammer deliberately, a person is saying that stammering can be acceptable and no longer needs to be hidden. We were also aware the client was telling us that he needed time to consider whether he was ready or even willing to take this step, and that we should give him the time he needed.

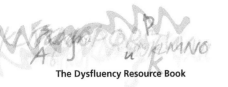

When to use

Voluntary stammering should not be introduced too early in therapy. The client needs to have completed the identification phase of therapy first and to have done some work on desensitisation, as suggested in the previous chapter. Desensitisation work is usually done alongside work on avoidance reduction.

We list here our reasons for regarding voluntary stammering as one of the most powerful desensitisation tools for people who stammer:

• It encourages people to approach stammering, not run away from it.

• It is a way in which someone who stammers can directly let people know that he stammers, rather than spend his speaking turn in dread that others might find out.

• The reality of people's predictions about stammering can be tested out. Being in control of stammering allows them to examine the reactions of others more objectively and calmly.

• People who stammer learn that they can have control over *when* they stammer, rather than feeling powerless as they wait for the stammer to occur.

• They also have control over *how* they stammer; they can do so in a controlled way rather than with struggle.

• They can have some control over how they *feel* about stammering.

How to teach voluntary stammering

1   The client either repeats (about three or four times if possible) or prolongs the first sound of a non-feared word (for example, 's, s, s, seaside' or 'sssssssseaside'). It is important for clients to use non-feared words as this helps retain control over their speech. Clients may be advised to choose definite or indefinite articles, conjunctions, pronouns or other non information carrying words.

2   The repetition or prolongation is made slowly and deliberately. The aim is for the 'stammer' to be seen and heard by the listener.

3   It is useful if both the repetition and the prolongation type of voluntary stammering can be experimented with. Some clients prefer to use types of stammering that are least like their own, while other clients prefer to use methods which sound closer to their own pattern.

4   The client uses good eye contact with the listener. In this way he 'owns' his stammering and shows the listener that he is not trying to hide it. He can also monitor the listener's reaction more objectively.

5   The client should be encouraged to maintain an easy, relaxed posture. Some clients move their heads in time to the voluntary stammering iterations. This should be discouraged and the client encouraged towards a 'natural' production.

6   Initially, voluntary stammering should be used in the easiest situations for the client. This could be identified using a hierarchy (see Chapter 9 'Avoidance reduction therapy'; also the 'Avoidance' section in Chapter 6, p87). Gradually, the number of voluntary stammers that the client aims to carry out in these easy situations is increased. Over time voluntary stammering can be used more frequently and in more difficult situations.

7   The clinician should have a discussion with the client regarding the degree of openness that will accompany the voluntary stammering. It is useful for the client to experiment with not

telling others what he is doing and to judge their reaction. He should also be encouraged to tell some people in some situations and see if there is a different response.

Teaching voluntary stammering in the following way can help to reduce the anxiety that is sometimes created initially:

- It must be explained carefully, in great detail, with a proper rationale and as many times as necessary.

- Reading material should be given, so that clients can refer to this outside the therapy room and show it to significant others as appropriate. We use Handout 34 'Voluntary stammering' and also refer clients to self-help books, such as *To the Stutterer* (Stuttering Foundation of America, 1995) and *Self Therapy for the Stutterer* (Fraser, 2007), both available from the British Stammering Association (see 'References' for website).

- It is often crucial for significant others to understand the rationale behind voluntary stammering and to be prepared to play an active role in encouraging the client to use it. Without support and understanding from others, voluntary stammering can often feel just too difficult for clients to use.

- In group situations such as the ones we facilitate, there are members who are at different stages of therapy. We find the presence of the 'older' members invaluable in helping the newer ones to experiment with voluntary stammering, as they are able to talk about its benefits from a 'consumer's' viewpoint. Bringing in a former client to an individual or group therapy session can also be helpful. Group members can ask questions and have answers from a 'consumer' who they know understands because he too has experienced some of their doubts and fears about the approach.

- The clinician needs to be prepared to demonstrate voluntary stammering herself, so the client can see what the reality is like before he tries it.

- The client should use voluntary stammering in safe situations first, beginning with the therapy room, where any errors (for example, going too quickly, not maintaining eye contact) can be noted and changed in a 'safe haven'. He can then move on to using it with people with whom he feels at ease before approaching more difficult situations.

- Some clients feel more able to use voluntary stammering with those they know. Others prefer the anonymity of using it with strangers who they will never see again. Some may find it easier to first tell people what they are doing.

Common problems

In our experience, we have found that (with a little gentle persuasion) most clients are willing to have a go at voluntary stammering and many find it a helpful part of therapy which they keep in their 'tool box' when they leave (see Chapter 15 'Maintenance: a continuing process of change'). However, there are clients who find the whole process just too threatening and who would rather leave therapy than try it out. We do not think these clients should be coerced into using it; the benefits should be explained and they should try it in therapy, at least on a one-to-one basis, but if it creates too much anxiety, it is counter-productive to continue. The client may not yet be ready; he may never be ready.

Van Riper (1973) makes the point that 'pseudostuttering', as he calls it, should not be used indiscriminately, but for a specific purpose. He also suggests that some clients may use voluntary stammering 'to punish themselves masochistically or their listeners sadistically' (p287).

While we have not been aware of this in any of our clients, we feel it is a possibility to be aware of. Another way in which voluntary stammering can be abused, according to Van Riper, is through an exaggerated use of it, which can confirm the person's view that listeners react negatively to stammering.

It is important to stress to clients that voluntary stammering is not a technique leading to a cure and should not be thought of as such. It is not intended to improve the stammer; in fact, it is designed to increase it. However, there is often a hidden benefit to voluntary stammering, which is, ironically, a decrease in 'real' stammering. There are at least two possible reasons for this. One is that when stammering voluntarily, speech is inevitably slowed down somewhat. Another reason relates to one of the things commonly said about stammering: that it is what happens when you try not to stammer. When someone stammers deliberately, sometimes his 'real' stammering decreases because he is no longer as anxious about it, struggles less and gradually begins to feel he has more choices.

Activities *for voluntary stammering*

Discussion ⓘ ⚙
Introduce voluntary stammering using Handout 34 as a basis for discussion.

Demonstration ⓘ ⚙
The clinician (or a group member if available) demonstrates the process. This can be done inside the clinic, on the telephone and outside the clinic setting. Clients can discuss their feelings as observers and also watch to see how listeners react. It is important to be aware that even watching someone 'stammering' can feel unbearably difficult to some people who stammer and they may therefore need much preparation.

Practice ⓘ ⚙
With the clinician or in a pair with another group member, the client practises voluntary stammering in reading, speaking in a monologue or in conversation, at different places in the sentence (see the section titled 'Ideas for practising voluntary stammering', p124).
Places where it can be used include:

• on the first word of the sentence

• on the second word of the sentence

• on the last word of the sentence

• on the next word after a comma

• on every word

• on a specific sound

• on a cue from the clinician or another group member

• for a specified number of times.

It is probably a good idea to first of all discuss what the client should do if he fears genuine stammering in this practice session or if he actually does stammer. It may be necessary to adapt the exercise initially for some people to ensure that only non-feared words are voluntarily stammered on.

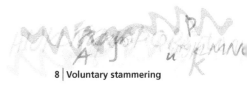
Hierarchy ⓘ Ⓖ

The client makes hierarchies (see Chapter 9 'Avoidance reduction therapy'; also the 'Avoidance' section in Chapter 6, p87) to determine the order in which he will introduce voluntary stammering. This can help to make the process feel more manageable.

Voluntary stammering competition Ⓖ

We sometimes find it helpful to introduce an element of competition into the use of voluntary stammering during the course of a group setting. Sometimes the competition is for individuals, at other times it is for teams to see who can get the highest score. We are frequently amazed at how some clients, who find it hard to use any voluntary stammering normally, will suddenly attain scores when they are competing. (We hasten to add that at *no other times* do we encourage our group clients to compete; indeed, we continually stress that therapy is about change at individual rates and in individual ways.)

Targets Ⓖ

Group members set themselves a number of voluntary stammers they must use during the course of a session. This must always be at least one more than in the previous session. If the target is not achieved there is a forfeit to be paid. Usually, this is in the form of a fine, but it can be an action or a gift. Some ideas we have used are listed below.

- Group members pay 1p for each stammer they have set themselves and failed to achieve. For example, if the target is 20 over the session and they achieve only 10, they pay 10p. The fine can be varied: it may be more or it may be a fixed rate if a person does not achieve their target. We give our fines to the British Stammering Association.

- The person who has achieved the least voluntary stammers has to buy a chocolate bar for the person who has achieved the most.

- Any person who has not achieved their target is made to say a nursery rhyme, do 20 sit-ups, sing a song or perform some other humiliating action!

These penalties can be adapted for use in individual therapy.

Home-based activity 1

The client underlines in a magazine or newspaper non-feared words on which to practise voluntary stammering. He does this while looking in a mirror, so that he confronts head on the thing he fears.

Home-based activity 2

The client tries the same exercise as above, but this time with someone listening.

Home-based activity 3

The client introduces voluntary stammering on non-feared words while talking to someone with whom he feels at ease. He starts with just one or two stammers and gradually increases his daily target, using his hierarchy to extend his use of voluntary stammering into increasingly difficult areas. We suggest that people do not keep their daily target too low. The reason is that often this is counter-productive, as the anxiety involved in doing each stammer remains just as high each time if there is a big gap between attempts.

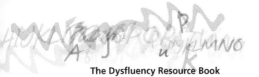

Ideas for practising voluntary stammering

The client is instructed to use voluntary stammers at a specific point in the sentence (see 'Practice' activity , p122).

Reading

The language may be kept quite simple here as reading is most likely to be used in order to familiarise the client with the technique. The target word on which the client is to use voluntary stammering can be underlined.

It is so cold today.

My dog is getting really fat.

The park is very near my house.

Have you seen what she is wearing?

She has just bought some new curtains.

Can I have two packets of those sweets, please?

Are you having a holiday this year?

I went to a great restaurant the other day.

What is your favourite type of food?

Do you like walking?

I love the look of that house.

That picture has not been put up straight.

His teacher is leaving at the end of term.

Supper is nearly ready.

His favourite colour is purple.

Their friends are emigrating to New Zealand.

Why do you think they chose that colour scheme?

Our newspaper gets delivered at the same time every day.

I am changing my phone.

You stayed in a lovely hotel.

Monologue

Topics can be increasingly emotive and/or complex as the client gets used to the technique and can cope with executing the task as well as thinking about the content of his speech.

Talk about:

Your favourite film

The month of the year you like most/least

The country you would most like to visit

A great meal you have eaten/cooked recently

What you like to do in the evenings

People in your family

Your best friend

A teacher you liked/disliked

An embarrassing moment

Something that really annoys you

Something you would save if there was a fire

A habit you have broken/not broken.

Conversation

Again, the complexity of the content can be developed over time. The client talks with a partner or the clinician, asking and answering questions on the following topics:

A holiday you have enjoyed

The sort of clothes you like to wear

A book you will always remember

Your dream car

What you take on holiday

Your favourite sort of TV programme

Speech therapy you received as a child

Things you enjoyed as a child

A friend you have lost touch with

When you lost something important

Things that wind you up

What you feel about capital punishment

Times you have been teased

Things you would never do

What you would do if you had the courage.

Voluntary stammering

Voluntary stammering is exactly what it sounds like: it is stammering on purpose. It is not a new idea, but a tried and tested procedure. In fact, therapists have been aware of its value since the 1930s. It is important not to think of voluntary stammering as a technique, but as a part of desensitisation. Your therapy so far should have helped you to feel a little less anxious about your stammer and other people's reaction to it. Voluntary stammering will extend this process and show you that you are able to stammer and feel in control. It is *not* meant to make you more fluent; in fact, it is designed to make you stammer more. It is meant to help you feel differently about stammering, and about yourself when you stammer.

Why should I stammer deliberately?

There are several reasons for suggesting what we realise must sound like a very strange idea:

1   When you stammer voluntarily, you are stammering under control. It is a very deliberate act, designed to help you stammer in a new way. You are no longer the passenger; instead you take the steering wheel.

2   Using this technique, you have choices.

  • You decide *when* to stammer. Many people who stammer spend a lot of their fluent speaking time worrying about when they will stammer and be 'caught out'. By using voluntary stammering, *you* can decide when to let the listener know that you stammer and as a result you may well find you enjoy the rest of the conversation more. You can pay more attention to *what* you are saying, rather than whether your listener will find out about the stammer.

  • You decide *how* you stammer. You learn that you do not have to respond to stammering with struggle and tension, but can stammer in a calm and controlled way. Later on in therapy you will find this helpful if you go on to modify your actual stammer.

  • You will also find that you can choose *how* you feel about stammering. The process enables you to stammer without experiencing so much of the fear or other negative emotions which so often accompany stammering.

3   By deciding to stammer, you are being open and honest about your speech. You are telling the listener that you stammer. You are more able to be the 'real you'.

4   When you stammer under control, because you do it with good eye contact, you can see how your listener is responding and be more objective about his reaction.

5   Voluntary stammering is the opposite of avoidance. Instead of running away from the stammer, you go towards it. You no longer need to hide it.

What should I do when I stammer voluntarily?

- Stammer on the first sound of the word. Either repeat the sound several times, for example, 't, t, t, tea' (sometimes called a 'bounce') or prolong the sound (sometimes called a 'slide') as with 'sssssssea'. Try to use both sorts of stammering. Some sounds are less easy to prolong, for example, plosive sounds like 'd' and 'b'. You will need to be taught how to soften these first.

- Stammer voluntarily on a word where you would not anticipate your usual stammer occurring. Often people find it helpful to choose words which are not very important to the meaning of the sentence, such as 'the' or 'and'. Words in the middle of a sentence can be better for some people to use than the first word. Do not use voluntary stammering on a word that starts with one of your feared sounds.

- Look at the person you are talking to. The aim is to learn to feel comfortable about stammering and to be able to assess the listener's reaction as objectively as possible.

- Stammer slowly and deliberately. Remember, the idea is to show the stammer, not to rush through it and try to hide it.

- Use voluntary stammering initially in a relaxed situation. You may prefer to try it out at first when reading out loud alone or with someone you feel comfortable with. Later on, you may choose to use it in more difficult situations.

- Some people find it helpful to explain to their listener what they are doing, some do not. You can experiment by telling some and not others, and seeing what difference it makes to you.

- Try not to move your head or body when you stammer deliberately; maintain a relaxed posture.

What if I start to really stammer?

Sometimes people are concerned that a voluntary stammer will turn into a real one and they will lose control. If you follow the instructions above this is less likely to occur. Most problems happen because people stammer too quickly or stammer on a feared word. If, however, a real stammer occurs, aim to stay as calm as you can. This, too, can be a useful desensitisation tool.

How often should I use voluntary stammering?

Start off by using just a few voluntary stammers until you feel you are doing them correctly. As you feel more confident, you can increase both the number you use and also introduce them gradually into increasingly difficult situations. After that, the sky's your limit!
Many people find that they continue to use voluntary stammering long after they leave therapy. Others only find it helpful for a relatively short period. You can decide what is best for you.

Routledge
Taylor & Francis Group

9 | Avoidance reduction therapy

Bryng Bryngelson, Wendell Johnson and Charles Van Riper, known collectively as the Iowa movement, were among the first to discuss the importance of reducing avoidance behaviours in adults who stammer. However, Joseph Sheehan and, after his death, his wife Vivian are most associated with this approach. Sheehan wrote extensively for two decades about avoidance in the context of his Conflict Theory in which he related stammering to the avoidance of speaking. He argued that stammering was the result of two opposing urges: the urge to speak (the approach response) and the desire to hold back from speaking (the avoidance response). He believed that this theory helped individuals to understand the relationship between their anxiety and stammering. He was also of the view that any treatment regarded as effective in the long term should target reduction of these avoidance behaviours. For Sheehan, avoidance reduction was the only form of therapy required to treat adults who stammered. However, his therapy was challenging and directly addressed fundamental issues, including how the individual construed himself. Sheehan wrote:

> two kinds of acceptance are asked of the stutterer. First, he must develop sufficient acceptance of himself as a stutterer to stop concealing the problem from himself and others – long enough to undertake a systematic weakening of the handicapping behaviours via principles of learning. Second, he must accept the goal of less than perfect fluency, for no one has that. In some cases, those with a history of lifelong stuttering are going to continue to show more than the usual amount of dysfluency. To plan otherwise is to deny experience and to court disaster.
> (1979, p178)

We concur with Sheehan that avoidance reduction is a principal component of therapy and advocate that most clients work on this area. For many of our clients, avoidance reduction and the resulting behaviour of open stammering is a liberating experience and can be the start of a new way of managing stammering.

In his approach–avoidance conflict theory Sheehan identified several distinct levels of avoidance:

Word level. At this level there are conflicting urges to approach or to avoid speaking feared words. Some clinicians in the UK subdivide this level into sound and speech avoidance (Logan & Sheasby, 2007). Clinically, clients presenting with word avoidance will substitute one word for another, which may be related or unrelated to the original target word (for example, 'Are we going to go out for an Indian meal tonight?' where 'curry' has been substituted by 'Indian

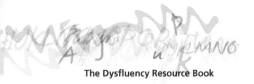
meal'). Where it is an unrelated word, the substitution may also require the speaker to reconstruct the rest of the sentence in order to clarify his intended meaning (for example, 'Are we going out for something to eat tonight? I mean shall we eat at that place we went to with your sister?'). If the word is significantly different in meaning the speaker will have to perform some 'verbal gymnastics' to make it fit, or can end up communicating an entirely different message. Consequently, some individuals with marked word avoidance use circumlocutions and/or reorder words in sentences.

Situation level. Sheehan defined this level as avoidance of specific situations involving communication and some degree of social interaction. Avoidance at this level can be confined to one situation in particular, for example, using the telephone or ordering at a bar or in a restaurant, but usually it is more generalised. It can also be quite subtle, with individuals rationalising their behaviour with such excuses as 'I didn't really need to go there' and justifying their actions to themselves rather than confronting their avoidance. Systematic situation avoidance is seen by some experts as the beginning of significant compromise in an individual's life.

Feelings. This level is defined as the avoidance of expressing feelings such as anger, upset, intimacy. The avoidance may be linked to one particular emotion, such as expressing gratitude. Some people may avoid several emotions and may appear lacking in feeling as a result. Some individuals who stammer have said that the expression of emotion is 'letting their guard down' and 'letting the stammer out'.

Relationships. The avoidance of issues relating to relationships would initially include making new friends, which involves initiating conversations, introducing oneself to others, actively placing oneself in contexts where social interactions take place, for example, going to parties and meeting people at venues such as pubs, sporting events and leisure clubs. Later, other behaviours would be required to build and develop the relationship, such as creating dialogue, asking and answering questions, imparting information (often relating to oneself). Finally, in order to maintain the friendship, individuals need to take responsibility to follow up contacts (for example, by telephoning) and may have a role in affirming and supporting others. All of these types of behaviours would be avoided at relationship level.

Self role. This is defined as the avoidance of accepting oneself as a person who stammers. The person does not live harmoniously with his stammer and does all he can to hide it from others. He makes negative predictions about stammering: 'If people know I have a stammer they will think I am inferior, unconfident, unintelligent' and so on. His avoidances at all the other levels may be high as a consequence. In his attempts to flee from the self who stammers, he is intent on pursuing the elusive fluent self, which he may feel to be his only solution.

When to use

- With clients with significant levels of avoidance at all levels and little overt stammering behaviour, sometimes called interiorised stammering (Douglas & Quarrington, 1952).

- With clients who demonstrate significant areas of avoidance in one or more of Sheehan's levels.

- After work on identification of stammering behaviour and covert issues, including avoidances (see Chapter 6 'Covert identification'), has been carried out.

- Alongside desensitisation activities.

- With more severe stammerers, alongside elements of speech control. More severe stammerers may not feel able to work on avoidance, knowing that it is likely to increase their stammering, without some means of controlling their speech.

Common problems

Although we list the activities in terms of each of Sheehan's avoidance levels, we are aware that the different levels are frequently intertwined and so, in effect, several levels are often being worked on at once. It is also apparent that when someone sets out to reduce one level of avoidance, they inevitably notice that other levels are involved. For example, in working on the situation avoidance of not travelling on a bus, the person realises it is the destination which he has to say and the fear of stammering in front of a colleague which are also problems.

It is sometimes assumed that Sheehan's levels are hierarchical, with word and situational levels easier to tackle than self role. However, there is no evidence in Sheehan's work that the levels were meant to be interpreted in this way. Therefore it is important not to pre-empt a hierarchy of difficulty for these levels; always ask the client.

Activities for reduction of word avoidance

Cancelling out word avoidance 🛈 ⚙

The aim of this activity is for the person to counteract his avoidance of a word as soon as he can. This will prevent fear of particular words from developing. As soon as a client realises that he has avoided words, he must work them back into the conversation. This can be done in different ways. One option is to adopt a completely honest approach, for example, 'I really meant to say "xxxx", but I thought I might stammer so I said "yyyy" instead'. This method has the added advantage of simultaneously working on desensitisation by being open about stammering.

In a situation where a person has tried to disguise his avoidance by pretending to have forgotten a word, he might say, 'I've remembered now, it was "xxxx"'. In some situations another alternative could be to say, 'I've changed my mind, I'd like "xxxx", not "yyyy"'.

Confronting the fear 🛈 ⚙

A client is asked to list those words he is most likely to avoid. The clinician (or other group members) asks him questions designed to elicit responses that contain the feared words. In such an exercise a client may find that by confronting words he has habitually avoided, he does not always stammer as badly as he feared, and maybe not at all.

Another version is for a client to be asked to say those difficult words spontaneously in either an individual or group session, or at home. For example, in the middle of an unrelated activity a clinician or group member or partner may ask, 'What is your name/address/phone number?', 'What do you call your speech problem?', 'How much is your bus fare?'

A further variation is for clients to telephone each other and ask for such information, in effect replicating a real-life situation an individual might face.

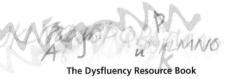

Just practise ⓘ ⓖ

Some clients find it helpful to practise lists of 'difficult' words, alone, in a group session or with significant others, in order to 'lay the stammering ghost' these words can create.

Target setting ⓘ ⓖ

A client sets targets for the maximum number of words he can allow himself to avoid daily. In having to limit himself, he must consider carefully the relative merits of avoiding each word. It can often then begin to feel easier just to go ahead and say the word and risk stammering.

A variation is targeting specific avoided words. In this version a client sets a target for the number of usually avoided words he will include in his conversations during that day. He may then report his success on a daily or weekly basis to a significant other or group member.

Activities for reduction of situation avoidance

Small steps ⓘ ⓖ

Hierarchies are a useful way of looking at avoided situations and establishing how they may be confronted in a systematic way. Hierarchies break goals into graded steps and reduce the enormity of a task. Each step on the hierarchy is small, in order to build as a high degree of success as possible. Steps are practised until they can be carried out with a minimum of anxiety (see Handout 35 'Making a hierarchy'). In this activity a client identifies situations that he habitually avoids and lists the steps he might take in approaching such situations.

In working through such a hierarchy, the person sometimes finds that his goals change: for example, he may discover that it is no easier to make an internal call than an external one, or that the length of the call does not make it any harder. Hierarchies therefore need to be flexible; they should be modified in the light of experience.

As we mentioned earlier, it is important to be aware that hierarchies are individual; what is easier for one person may be harder for another, so clinicians should not make assumptions for the client.

Discussion ⓖ

In a group setting a client talks about a situation that he habitually avoids. Other group members help him identify a number of coping strategies he might use to help him approach the situation. This is a good way of looking at the difficulties that have kept individuals from approaching feared situations. Once coping strategies are developed, the person may feel more confident to 'have a go'.

If we take an example of going to book a train ticket, the ideas might include:

• go at a time when there are less likely to be crowds

• explain you have a stammer and may take longer to say what you need

• use good non-verbal communication, especially appropriate eye contact

• speak slowly

• use voluntary stammering

• thank the person for their help

• use any speech techniques you have learned which could be helpful

• don't judge success on whether you stammer but on if you achieve the task.

This activity can be used in individual therapy, but there are obviously fewer people involved to generate ideas. A client could be asked to discuss ideas at home and with friends and then bring them back to therapy.

Role play ⚙

Following on from the previous exercise, or as an independent activity, a client can explore different ways of tackling his avoidance in the safety of clinic by role playing his different options. As in any role play, it is important that a client not only experiments with different behaviour options, but also considers different ways of feeling and thinking.

Elaboration of the fear ⓘ ⚙

In order to tackle the root of the avoidance it is useful to explore with a client what he believes to be the underlying fear. This needs to be done in an atmosphere of calm acceptance and empathetic support. In a group setting it would be important to carry out such an activity when the group has established itself and support mechanisms are in place.

Consequences ⓘ ⚙

Sometimes a client can be so intent and focused on his avoidance that he has not considered the implications of continuing his behaviour. It is therefore useful for the clinician to engage in a discussion of the consequences of continuing situation avoidance for the client and also, equally important, for those significant others in his environment. For example, what would happen if the client continued to avoid using the telephone? He would not being able to speak to his family when he travelled away from home, or when they were away from him. He would not be able to phone for a taxi when public transport or his own transport was unavailable. He would not be able to phone for emergency services.

Activities for reduction of feelings avoidance

Elaborating an emotion ⓘ ⚙

When a client is not used to expressing a particular emotion he may struggle to know what it 'looks like'. He may be unfamiliar with the ways in which it can be expressed in words, or through expression or touch. In these instances it is beneficial for him first to discuss with a clinician or other group members how they might express this particular emotion. Alternatively, the client might be asked to gather data on how this emotion is expressed by others in different settings outside the clinic. This then forms the basis for him to explore the alternatives that are available to him.

Role plays ⚙

In this exercise a client is asked to identify a situation where he did not express an emotion that he wishes he had. The role play is carried out in two parts, first as the situation was, and then as the client would have liked it to be. In a group setting the person concerned can choose a 'cast' to play out the situation as it was. There are benefits either if the person plays himself (he gets it right) or casts someone else in the role (he sees it more objectively). Having played the scene, the group members discuss what happened, how those involved felt in their role and what changes might be made in the future. The scene is then replayed in the new way and discussed again in the light of the modifications made.

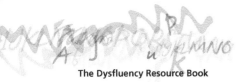
Home-based activity *Targeted emotions*[1]

In this activity the client selects emotions that he finds hard to express and targets the number of times he will try to express them over a given period. He is encouraged to write a full description of the event, his own feelings and others' reactions as soon as possible afterwards and to report back to the clinician and/or group. Use Handout 36 'Diary sheet for avoidance reduction exercises'.

Activities *for reduction of relationship avoidance*

How do relationships work? ⓘ ⚙

The clinician facilitates a discussion with the client or group of clients about key aspects of relationships.

- How are relationships formed?

- What are the important components of a close friendship?

- How are they maintained?

Developing roles ⓘ ⚙

Building on the discussion of the previous activity, the client takes an aspect that he wishes to develop. Experiments are then negotiated with the client for him to try out: for example, establishing relationships may require placing the client in situations where he meets new people. Establishing new relationships may require him to practise initiating speech (see Chapter 2 'Communication skills').

Role play ⚙

Role playing social events can be a way of learning strategies to employ in social situations. Sometimes relationships are avoided because a client lacks experience in making them. He may be unsure of how to go about starting, continuing and ending conversations because this is something he has not done to any great extent. Instead, he has hoped that someone else will take responsibility.

The following are ideas for role plays:

- Role playing a party situation may reveal that, for example, there is more than one way to be introduced. The person can not only approach someone 'cold' but might alternatively get to know people by taking drinks round or by specifically engineering it so that a mutual friend introduces him to someone new.

- If a client finds it hard to break into an ongoing conversation, a trios exercise can be used. Two people have a conversation and a third tries to become a part of what is going on. Useful and not so useful strategies can then be discussed.

- We are aware that some of our clients find small talk particularly difficult. Role play can be a useful way of trying out different tactics in a safe environment where failure does not matter. Using video can provide helpful feedback. Scenes we have used in this context include waiting at a bus stop or in a doctor's surgery, asking for information or buying something from a shop (see Chapter 2 'Communication skills').

---

[1] The tasks in this activity can follow on from each other in a sequence or be carried out separately.

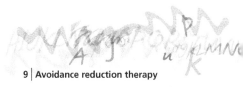

Discussions ⓘ ⚙

The clinician facilitates discussion around the pros and cons of issues associated with making and maintaining relationships. Here are some suggestions:

- Be proactive – seize the initiative rather than waiting for others to approach you.

- Express your feelings rather than pretending to agree and then feeling frustrated or aggrieved.

- Spend time trying to be fluent, ensuring the stammer is not seen, rather than explaining the problem and the difficulties it can create and enlisting the help of others.

- Keep quiet and run the risk of appearing bored or boring rather than saying the things you want to.

- Don't go out with friends because it puts too much pressure on your speech, but risk your friends thinking you don't want to meet with them.

Activities for reduction of self role avoidance

Sentence completion ⓘ ⚙

A client is given a written list of unfinished sentences to complete (see Handout 37 'Sentence completion exercise'). The sentences are completed individually and can be read out to the clinician in individual therapy or to the whole group. Answers are discussed and challenged with reference to the difficulties each client has in accepting himself as someone who stammers. For example, if the sentence 'People may think stammerers are ...' is completed with the word 'stupid', a client can be asked to estimate how many people might think this, what evidence he has for it and how valid that evidence is. If the client believes that many people think in this way, therapy must help him either change his own construing of the listener or look at ways in which he can challenge the listener's perception and/or provide an alternative construction to his own behaviour.

Elaborating self role ⓘ ⚙

The clinician discusses with the client what exactly someone who is at ease with their stammering would be like. It is useful to elaborate ideas under three main headings:

- cognitions or thoughts (for example, thinking about the moment and not anticipating stammering)

- feelings or emotions (for example, feeling content with communicating a specific message irrespective of the level of fluency)

- behaviours or actions (for example, being active in a conversation, asking questions and leading when appropriate).

Learning from others ⓘ ⚙

Having established the features of self role that are key to the client's construing (see the previous activity), the clinician asks an ex-client or someone still in therapy to demonstrate one of the key features, for example, open stammering. The clinician then facilitates a discussion on the advantages and disadvantages of this feature between the two individuals.

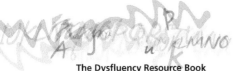

Fixed role therapy 🛈 ⚙️

The clinician discusses with the client how he might experiment with one or more of the key features of acceptance of stammering. They agree on how this 'experiment' might be carried out and how the client might behave, think and feel while carrying out this experimental role. In effect, the client is 'trying out' acceptance and acting 'as if' he did not have a particular feature of self role avoidance. Following the experiment, the client reports back on how it went and, with the clinician, determines if further experimentation in certain areas is required or if there are areas he could adopt on a more permanent basis.

Working with hierarchies 🛈 ⚙️

Hierarchies can be used to establish steps in certain aspects of self role, for example, telling people about stammering and/or speech and language therapy (see Handout 35 'Making a hierarchy').

Worst case scenario 🛈 ⚙️

The client describes his worst stammering scenario, real or imagined. Questions from the clinician and other clients help to tease out what the fears are about and what stammering represents for the client, for example, being inferior, being different, being undervalued.

Activity for considering avoidance ⚙️

Many quotations from Sheehan can be used for discussion topics in this area. Some may need modifying for the specific individual or group you are working with. We offer you just two for consideration.

> We have come to believe that stuttering is perpetuated by successful avoidance, by the successful suppression of outward stuttering behavior and the substitution of false fluency, or by inner patterns of fluency.
> (1983, p13)

> See how much of your iceberg you can bring up above the surface. When you reach the point where you're concealing nothing from yourself and from your listener, you won't have much handicap left. You can stutter yourself out of this problem of stuttering, if you do it courageously and openly.
> (1983, p6)

Making a hierarchy

Very often a task can seem enormous when looked at as a whole, but when it is broken down into its component parts, perhaps even with some kind of time scale attached to it, it can seem much easier. Take the example of decorating a room; transforming it from a shabby, uninspired area into a fresh looking modern one may seem a daunting task. When you look at it in a staged approach, however, it can become more manageable. You could, for example, decide to spend an evening looking at colour charts, mulling over curtain fabrics and wallpapers. After this you might move or cover the furniture. The next stage is perhaps to do the preparation, scraping off the wallpaper one evening, sanding down paintwork another, and on a third filling in the cracks, and so on … You get the idea!

Using a hierarchy as part of your therapy is similar. You may feel you could never manage to ask for fish and chips. If you take a staged approach you may find you can get there in the end. The stages to go through will differ for each individual but could, for example, involve some of the following: walking to the shop and standing by when someone else orders, saying 'hello' to the person who is serving and asking for something that is easier to say in an empty shop with someone supportive near at hand in case you panic. You can use a hierarchy to plan this sort of task. You can also employ a hierarchy to plan, say, the situations in which you will use voluntary stammering. This sort of a hierarchy might read as follows: alone when reading aloud, reading into a tape recorder, talking with your nearest and dearest, talking to a good friend, and so on, until you reach whatever it is that is the worst imagined scenario.

Things to remember when making and using hierarchies

1   Break down a task into small steps. Remember they are not set in tablets of stone; they must be flexible. For example, when you carry out an experiment, if you find step 2 is actually easier than step 1, then alter the order in which you attempt the steps. You can also skip steps if you feel they are too easy or add extra ones if you find there is too big a gap between them.

2   Using a hierarchy can give you a boost. Even if you do not reach your desired goal as quickly as you might like to, you can see yourself getting closer to it. You may still not be able to phone to make a complaint or order a complicated meal, but looking back over the steps you have taken in the hierarchy can show you have made some progress.

3   If you are going through a bad patch in your talking, you can use the hierarchy both to boost your confidence and to get you back on track. Sometimes you will feel your speech is back to square one, but when you look at hierarchies you have worked on you will often be able to see that you have not actually gone back as far as you thought. You can also identify an appropriate starting place for the work you have to do to bring yourself back on course.

Routledge
Taylor & Francis Group

Continued on Handout **35.2** ➜

H35.1

← Continued from Handout **35.1**

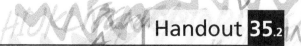

Sample hierarchy for reducing situation avoidance

Goal: to telephone a friend

Steps to be worked at in turn until each can be achieved without undue anxiety.

- Pick up the telephone.
- Say 'hello' while the dialling tone is sounding.
- Dial a number but put the phone down before it rings.
- Phone internally at the clinic and say 'hello'.
- Phone internally and say more.
- Prepare the friend for a one-word phone call.
- Make the above.

Continue to make calls to friend, increasing length, complexity of content or emotional level.

Routledge
Taylor & Francis Group

Diary sheet for avoidance reduction exercises

Day	Situation	Strategy used
Monday		
Tuesday		
Wednesday		
Thursday		
Friday		
Saturday		
Sunday		

Routledge
Taylor & Francis Group

Sentence completion exercise

Complete the following sentences. Your answers will be discussed in front of the clinician and/or group.

When the exercise has been completed, you may choose to discuss it with your friends and family.

People may think stammerers are ....

When I stammer at home people think I am ....

When I stammer with strangers I feel ....

When I stammer with friends I feel ....

Most people who stammer are the type of people who ....

Stammering in public places makes me feel ....

I'd rather..than stammer

My best friends think my stammer is ....

Stammering stops me from ....

If I didn't stammer, I would ....

Stammering as a child made me ....

I blame my stammer for ....

If I were to accept my stammer fully, I ....

Fluency would mean..

Fluent people are ....

This page may be photocopied for instructional use only. *The Dysfluency Resource Book* © J Turnbull & T Stewart 2010

10 | Relaxation

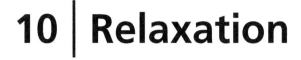

Relaxation approaches in one form or another have been associated with therapy for people who stammer for at least a century. It is understandable why this should be the case, as stammering is a communication disorder frequently characterised by struggle and tension. However, there is still no empirical evidence to suggest that, in isolation at least, relaxation is a strategy which has any long-lasting effect on stammering. Relaxation can be, and frequently is, induced in the safe haven of speaking situations in the clinic, sometimes with subsequent temporary positive effects on fluency, but once the client is outside the tension often remains very difficult to control.

Van Riper (1973) argued against the teaching of relaxation techniques, claiming that relaxation would instead emerge as a 'by-product' of the 'stammer more fluently' and avoidance reduction approaches. He said, 'it should come as the result of successful coping, not as the instrument for coping' (p284).

So why do we still include relaxation in this second edition of our book? Manning reminds us that 'being able to relax in the midst of life's many anxiety-producing stimuli is a valuable skill for anyone' (2000, p302). There is certainly evidence that being able to relax is associated with physiological changes, among them decreased heart and respiration rate, decreased blood pressure and an increase in alpha wave brain activity (Bourne, 2005). In addition, Bourne notes other benefits associated with relaxation, including reduced generalised anxiety, prevention of cumulative stress, increased productivity, energy levels and self-confidence. Although the ability to relax may not produce fluency for most people, for many it will make it easier to control the stress that speaking in difficult situations can bring about. Being more physically and mentally relaxed may also help an individual to put in place other techniques which aim to increase fluency, such as easy onset, soft contacts and block modification.

Historically, relaxation has more commonly been incorporated into a number of other therapeutic approaches, rather than used in isolation. It has, for example, been used in conjunction with systematic desensitisation (Brutten & Shoemaker, 1967), anxiety control training (Snaith, 1981), hypnosis (Greer, 1991) and more recently, mindfulness-based meditation (Cheasman, 2007).

When to use

Relaxation techniques are usually taught early in therapy, once identification has highlighted tension as a significant factor for the individual. Relaxation may be taught alongside desensitisation and, if required, before the teaching of breathing or speech modification, for which relaxation is a prerequisite.

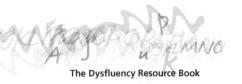
Types and uses of relaxation

1 *Tension control* is used to monitor and reduce the amount of muscle tone needed for a particular behaviour, to make sure that the amount of effort matches that required for the activity. *Progressive relaxation* is a useful approach here as it helps a person to become aware of sites of muscle tension. This involves going through groups of muscles in turn, tensing and then releasing tension. It is recommended that clinicians develop a style and a form which feels natural and comfortable and with which they are happy, but readers may initially want to use the suggested script given in Handout 38 'Progressive relaxation'.

Possible problems with progressive relaxation

- People may get cramps when tensing: the person needs to stop as soon as they occur. If cramps occur regularly, this may suggest unsuitability for progressive relaxation.

- Some people find this process makes them laugh, usually out of embarrassment, especially when they are 'pulling faces' during relaxation of facial muscles. Laughter is often associated with a letting go of stress and usually subsides with continued practice.

2 *Stress control* uses relaxation to manage situations in which an individual finds it difficult to cope with the tension associated with anxiety and stress. *Systematic desensitisation* is a helpful approach for such a client. Using this technique, the client learns a basic relaxation technique and then applies it to control anxiety, initially in imagined situations and then transferring to real life. (We suggest that clinicians wanting to learn this technique download 'Anxiety control training 1' on the *Living Life to the Full* website cited in the section 'Anxiety control training' on p148.)

Relaxation methods that can be used include (1) quick relaxation techniques, (2) shorter 'time out' relaxation tasks, and (3) deep relaxation (usually taking considerably longer), which incorporates muscle relaxation, cognitive processing, visualisation and suggestion.

Possible problems with systematic desensitisation

- Some clients may have a fear of relaxing and for some, putting trust in another person can bring about a feeling of loss of control. This can be helped by the clinician's use of language, for example, telling the client to be 'as relaxed as you want to be', and phrasing instructions as possibilities: 'Your left arm may relax more than your right arm or your right arm more than your left, I don't know'.

- The client is unwilling to practise at home: if this is the case it is likely that the clinician has either not explained the benefits adequately or the client does not feel this sort of approach is right for him. There is then little point in proceeding.

- The client is unable to practise at home: sometimes circumstances prevent the time and space for this sort of practice. For example, there may not be a room available, the phone keeps ringing, or other people or children make demands on the person's time. This may be a particular problem if the client has not been open about his stammering and therapy and therefore feels unable to express his need for time and quiet. If the obstacles cannot be overcome, it may be best not to work on full relaxation but to give the client techniques he can use 'on the spot'.

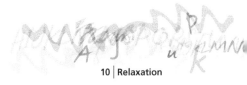
In our clinics we have used relaxation exercises in both group and individual therapy sessions. In these instances a client feels the need to have some means of coping with high levels of anxiety and accompanying tension before being able to work on other aspects such as avoidance or speech techniques. It appears that the tension and often panic disable him from concentrating on other factors and he needs at least to feel he can manage this first.

How to teach deep relaxation

There are several aspects to consider when practising and teaching deep relaxation.

The environment

Before embarking on the teaching of relaxation, the clinician must consider the environment in which the client is to learn to relax. The reality is that many of us, unfortunately, do not work in clinic settings which are conducive to relaxation; they are often noisy rooms, contain distracting features, and may be shared with other professionals and therefore contain equipment of various types, and so on. In these circumstances, we have to do the best we can. The following are some points to consider before the client comes into the room.

- Try to ensure the room is at a comfortable temperature. It is easier to relax in a room that is too warm rather than too cold. Draughts should be minimised where possible.

- Endeavour to prevent interruptions. It is a good idea to place a 'Do not disturb' notice on the door before the session starts. Telephones should be switched to 'divert' where possible or taken off the hook, and receptionists and secretaries should be informed that interruptions are to be prevented. Should any interruptions occur, the therapist should deal with them in a calm way, while instructing the client to concentrate on their breathing and not the interruption. (We have managed to continue a session this way when a non-urgent fire alarm was ringing!)

- Reduce the brightness of the light in the room where possible by closing curtains or blinds, or dimming/switching off lights.

- Reduce distractions. Where there are permanent features in the clinic that cannot be removed, the client's chair or place allocated for relaxation should be situated away from these features and away from any windows. Most clients are happy to close their eyes during a relaxation session, but there are those who prefer to keep them open throughout.

- It is also worth alerting colleagues who may be working in adjacent rooms that a relaxation session is taking place so they can be mindful and monitor the level of their interactions.

Preparing the client

It can be helpful for clients to plan to arrive a few minutes early and sit quietly in reception as a preparation for the session. Once in the clinic room, the client should have time to settle down before beginning the relaxation exercises. There may be issues on his mind that he needs to express before he can concentrate adequately.

The structure of the relaxation exercise should be explained fully to the client at the beginning of the session so he knows what to expect and what is required of him. In particular, we mention how to deal with extraneous noise, whether or not the client wishes to close his eyes and if any verbal responses will be required of him during the session.

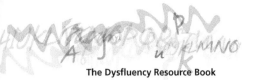

Comfort and positioning of the client are very important. He must be comfortable and any excess layers of clothes should be removed and tight clothes loosened. Regarding positioning, there are a number of reclining chairs on the market that are ideally suited to inducing relaxation. However, these are expensive and it is quite possible to use ordinary chairs or the floor. In the case of the floor, if there is no carpet, a blanket, rug or camping mat may prove useful. In some ways we feel that a normal chair, preferably with arm rests, is perfectly adequate, especially once a client has started to learn how to relax, as it demonstrates to the client that relaxation is not dependent on great comfort.

Preparing yourself as therapist

Make sure you are comfortable, warm and at ease. Try to clear your head of intrusive thoughts and use the session to relax yourself too!

Giving instructions

The tone of your voice and pacing of instructions can be helpful to the induction of relaxation. Speak slowly and clearly, using a calming voice. It is not necessary to keep your pitch and intonation flat and there is no need to whisper; clients need to hear what you say and should not have to struggle to follow your instructions.

Insert good pauses between instructions. Give the client time to monitor his muscle tone/ tension or imagine what you are asking him to do. If you carry out the activity in parallel with him once or twice, then, generally, you can get an idea of appropriate timing. However, remember that everyone is different and you may need to check that the pace is appropriate. Emphasise that the client is monitoring, reducing or controlling tension for himself. This is not something you are doing to him.

Monitoring your client

Once the relaxation is under way, how will you know your client is starting to relax? The following are possible guides. Some of these can be observed; others will only be clear after discussion with the client at the end of the session.

- 'Weight' of limbs: limbs should feel heavy.

- Muscle tone: muscle should feel soft, not hard.

- Heart rate: clinicians may be able to visually observe the client's heart rate (by the pulse in the neck) at the beginning and compare it with observations throughout the session.

- Respiration rate: clinicians should observe the client's rate of respiration at the start of the session and then again after about five or six minutes. It should be significantly slower and shallower.

- Eye movements: clinical experience has shown that more relaxed clients have fewer eye movements, both when the eyes are open and behind the lids when they are closed. The exception to this is during a task that requires some visualisation by the client; eye movements usually increase during this type of activity.

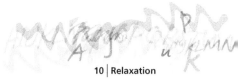

Winding down

Towards the end of any session involving relaxation the client should be forewarned that the exercise is coming to a close. The clinician can simply say:

> In a moment I am going to bring this session to an end by counting back from 6 to 1. When I reach 1 all feelings of heaviness will have gone, but the feelings of relaxation will remain. Counting back now … 6, 5, 4, lighter and lighter now, 3, 2 and 1.

The client should be given time to open his eyes, stretch and readjust his position.

Getting feedback

As we have said previously in this section, it is important to obtain feedback from the client on particular aspects of the session.

- The environment: how was the client's general comfort and ability to cope with any distractions?

- The relaxation position: was the position comfortable, did he manage to relax all muscle groups?

- The instructions and pacing: did he understand what was asked of him, was he given enough time to think and monitor, would he have liked the pace to be slower or faster?

- The level of relaxation attained: how relaxed did he feel, were there any areas in his body where he remained tense?

- If visualisation was used: what suggestions worked best, what were the relaxing images used by the client?

This information is essential to ensure the relaxation is tailor-made for the individual client and can then be adjusted to ensure his needs are met in future sessions.

'On the spot' techniques

These techniques are quick and easy to use in situations when a person needs some instant tension relief. In order to be effective such techniques should:

- be flexible enough to be used in a variety of situations

- not be obvious to others

- aid the person to feel *more* relaxed while carrying on with the task in hand.

Payne (1995) suggests that techniques for 'on the spot' exercises may be taken from any of the following approaches:

- physical actions

- scanning

- breathing

- cognitive changes.

We list some of Payne's suggestions below.

Releasing tension by physical actions

Key changes. These are specific actions the person can use to unlock patterns of tension.

1 Spreading the fingers: make the fingers and thumbs long, hold for a moment, stop, allow them to recoil back into a gently curved position.

2 Separating the teeth: drag the jaw downwards, feel the jaw hang down in the mouth, stop, feel the throat slacken, the tongue loosen and the lips gently touch.

3 Pulling the shoulders towards the feet: feel a distance increasing between the shoulders and the ears, stop and let the shoulders rest.

4 Pushing the head back: the shoulders are pulled down, the head is lifted, then carried up and back, keeping the chin pointed towards the feet. Stop in a comfortable position.

Posture. Good posture is important for releasing tension.

1 Tell yourself to 'think tall'.

2 Stretch parts of the body, for example the spine, which may have been held in a particular position for quite a while.

3 'Shaking a sleeve down': this looks quite natural and can loosen arm and shoulder muscles.

4 'Chin on a shelf': imagine placing your chin on a shelf which is directly in front of you, thereby lifting the chin and aiming to balance the head on the spinal column.

Additional ideas for posture can be found in Chapter 2 'Communication skills'.

Releasing tension by scanning

This involves scanning the body for sites of tension, as if doing a short form of a relaxation exercise.

1 Relaxation by recall with counting: two counts are given to four groups of muscles: 1… 2… (arms relax) 3… 4… (head and neck relax) 5… 6… (trunk relaxes) 7… 8… (legs relax) 9… 10… (whole body relaxes).

2 Behavioural relaxation checklist: work through a list of ten postures that release tension, for example, loose throat, dropped shoulders.

3 Sweeping the body: sweep the body with an imaginary soft paintbrush.

4 The ripple: a ripple effect relaxation begins at the head and rolls through the body to the feet, relaxing each part of the body in turn.

Releasing tension by breathing

Slowing the breathing rate can counteract the effect of the physiological arousal brought about by the action of the parasympathetic nervous system. Payne (1995) makes three suggestions:

1 use of abdominal breathing for a quietening effect

2 using words as cues: repetition of words associated with relaxation, for example, 'relax', 'calm'

3 a breathing cycle: taking a deeper, slower in-breath, holding it and slowly letting it out again. Pause before repeating to avoid hyperventilation.

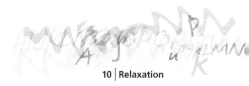

In addition, we like the idea, often taught in antenatal classes, whereby the person imagines the breath entering their body at the top of the head, travelling all the way through the body, in all the muscle groups, and leaving the body through the ends of the toes.

Cognitive strategies

These are described as ways of dealing with stress by changing thought. Suggestions include:

- self-talk: for example, 'I am in control' (we feel it is best if the actual phrase is chosen by the client and therefore more personally meaningful to him)

- imagery: for example, imagining oneself as being like a rag doll

- thinking of a smile or a positive moment (for example, a good experience or happy occasion).

Finally in this section, we would like to share another quick cognitive relaxation strategy we have found useful, especially before something we perceive will be stressful. As you breathe deeply in and out (to a count of however many you feel comfortable with), say to yourself:

> MIND AWAKE AND ALERT
> BODY CALM AND RELAXED
> I AM NOT GOING TO LET THIS BOTHER ME
> Smile in your mind as you say the words.
> (Source unknown)

Because a person who stammers may feel stress particularly in his face, head and neck, we have included some exercises specifically for these areas on Handout 39 'Techniques for head and neck relaxation'. It is best to show the client exactly how to do these exercises first and practise with him in the clinic, rather than giving him the handout 'cold'.

We mentioned 'mindfulness-based meditation' near the start of this chapter. This approach helps a person to focus more on the moment and gradually to let go of emotions such as shame, which are frequently associated with the past. We do not propose to describe this kind of therapy in detail in this chapter, as relaxation is not its main aim but rather an associated benefit. Cheasman (2007) outlines three benefits of this approach for people who stammer.

1 Acceptance: mindfulness meditation teaches acceptance of the self and the experience as opposed to struggle and avoidance of the experience. Cheasman refers to this not as resignation but as a radical change of relationship with the experience.

2 Awareness: the approach encourages the development of a non-judgmental observer stance in relation to thoughts about and reactions to stammering.

3 Calmness and relaxation: Cheasman stresses that mindfulness is not a relaxation technique, but that the development of a calm and relaxed relationship with stammering will be beneficial.

Readers interested in learning more about this approach are directed to the following texts: Kabat-Zinn, 1994; Segal *et al*, 2002; Cheasman, 2007.

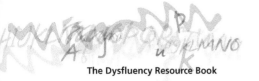
Anxiety control training (ACT)

ACT was devised as a discrete programme by Snaith (1974) but has its roots in three areas: cognitive behavioural therapy (CBT), hypnosis and autogenic training. In recent years there has been some controversy over the use of techniques such as ACT, which are aimed at helping a person control anxiety once it has occurred but not to look at the factors involved in maintaining the anxiety. The 'new generation' of cognitive therapists (see Beck *et al*, 1985; Borkovec & Costello, 1993; Wells, 1995) advocate instead that therapy should be geared towards disconfirming the beliefs responsible for the anxiety. They argue that teaching methods of control reinforces the belief that something bad can happen if you do not control it. In essence, then, behavioural therapies encourage a person to be vigilant so that he can be ready to use techniques to control his anxiety. Cognitive therapies undermine the beliefs that make a person feel control is needed. We feel the development of this approach is very exciting and our limited experience of working in this way has shown it to be helpful to our clients. However, we still find that ACT has much to offer, particularly for a client who needs to have a safety net for when his anxiety occurs or for the client who is not willing or able to work along purely cognitive lines. For some of our clients, ACT has been a turning point to greater feelings of control.

This perspective is also one proposed by Chris Williams, Senior Lecturer in Psychiatry at the University of Glasgow. He uses a cognitive behavioural therapy approach in his work and on his self-help website www.livinglifetothefull.com. This can be accessed free of charge by clients and clinicians. The website was set up to teach life skills, including recognising and changing unhelpful thoughts and behaviours, coping with depression, using assertiveness skills and problem solving. Of particular relevance to this chapter are two downloadable audio recordings of ACT, which Williams clearly sees as compatible with a CBT approach. The first is a relaxation induction and the second is on the introduction of anxiety and its control into the session. A client with a home computer can use this for home practice.

When to use

We do not use ACT with a dysfluent client who just becomes anxious in speaking situations; desensitisation and perhaps some general relaxation exercises are more appropriate in this context. We reserve ACT for a client who experiences anxiety in other aspects of his life, both in speaking and non-speaking situations. A person may also have specific anxieties, perhaps a particular fear or phobia, or a social anxiety; sometimes a client may just be a worrier or find it impossible to relax. Another individual can find it difficult to work on speech until he has reduced his anxiety levels. Gaining control over such anxiety is obviously positive in itself; it also 'clears the decks' for such a person to focus on his speech.

In order to ascertain if ACT may be useful for a particular client, both subjective and objective assessments can be used. On the subjective level, a client can be asked if he considers himself to be anxious or worries a lot or has any problems other than stammering. In addition, the person has to want to control his anxiety and be prepared to regularly practise the skill. Objectively, we use the Hospital Anxiety and Depression (HAD) scale (Zigmond & Snaith, 1983). This scale takes only a few minutes to complete and is scored as quickly. Two sub-scores are calculated, one for anxiety and one for depression. There are cut-off points where anxiety or depression are felt to be of some significance; the higher someone scores above these points, the more anxious or depressed he is likely to be. The depression score is also useful diagnostically as we would be unlikely to suggest ACT for use with a significantly depressed person. The technique relies on self-reinforcement, which tends to be difficult for a depressed client. The scale can be repeated at various points in therapy to ascertain how successful it is in treating the anxiety. It is essential that the client commits to practising the technique daily, if possible twice daily.

In our experience, ACT has been helpful to many of our clients. Benefits include:

• experiencing a greater sense of control over anxiety

• having more awareness of when anxiety starts and a feeling that it does not have to develop

• developing a higher threshold for anxiety.

How to teach anxiety control training

ACT usually involves between 10 and 15 sessions, each lasting about 15–20 minutes. The first three or four of these are taken up with teaching progressive relaxation and introducing visual imagery (a suggested form of words is in Snaith, 1981). The imagery in the first session is usually quite concrete and specific: a flower, for example. In the next and subsequent sessions the person is asked to think of a calm scene. What constitutes this will vary from person to person and the clinician should give the client freedom to think of something that represents personal calm and relaxation. Many of our clients use a seaside or countryside scene, sometimes familiar to them, sometimes drawn from their imagination. Others use a familiar room or a plant. Some use more abstract forms such as shapes or patterns.

After each of these initial sessions the client gives the clinician feedback on the following:

• the degree of relaxation achieved

• visual imagery experienced

• any difficulty in relaxing specific body areas (the clinician can offer more help with these areas at the next session)

• sensory feedback – warmth, tingling, heaviness and so on (signs of the client being relaxed and getting in tune with his body).

The clinician, too, notes things that may give clues as to the degree of relaxation experienced. These include stillness, lack of agitation, swallowing or throat clearing and deep relaxed breathing.

Once the client is able to achieve a good degree of relaxation in his practice at home, anxiety imagery is introduced, first into the clinical sessions and then into the home practice. In the first of these sessions the client is asked to think of himself in a scene that makes him feel 'just a little bit' anxious. He is asked to stay in the scene in his imagination and signal to us, perhaps by moving a finger, that he has done so. We often note physical signs of anxiety at this stage, perhaps a faster respiration rate or some general movement. In the next session we repeat this activity but give the client a 'coping mechanism' for dealing with the anxiety. This may be a specific word or set of words chosen by the client (such as 'calm down', 'take it easy', 'take control') and/or the instruction to take three or four deep, calming breaths. In subsequent sessions the format is the same. We do not work on a hierarchy of difficult situations (the list could be endless); rather we help people gain a sense of mastery over their anxiety in general. However, we do suggest the client works on scenes that cause him only low anxiety initially and then increases the amount of anxiety he learns to control over the weeks ahead.

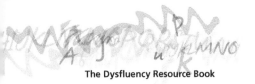
Possible problems

- The client does not put in the required practice. This may be for a number of reasons: his circumstances have changed and no longer allow it, other people are not co-operating in giving him the time and space he needs, or he finds he does not believe the technique will work. If discussion does not resolve these problems it is best to abandon ACT and resume if things change in the future.

- The person becomes depressed during the course of therapy. Again, it is best to avoid this kind of therapy until the depression has reduced.

- The person cannot experience anxiety in the clinical or home practice session. This may be because he is concerned about his ability to control it and therefore is not able to take the risk. He should be told to think only of low anxiety scenes until his confidence grows.

- The person is unable to gain control of the anxiety. This may be because ACT is a new skill which needs practice or because he is thinking of something which is too high in anxiety.

- The person's first imagined scene is one of high anxiety.

- Distracters: the person is unable to prevent distractions occurring, for example, the phone ringing, noise outside, other people interrupting.

Progressive relaxation

The aim of progressive relaxation is for you to recognise tension in your body and be able to release it. Once you learn to do this in your own practice sessions, you will start to be able to recognise tension – and release it – in your everyday life.

What to do

You can do this exercise in any position you choose: sitting, lying down or even standing. With each muscle group the process is the same: tighten the muscles for several seconds and then release them.

- Start with your feet. Curl the toes of one foot up and feel the tension. Let go and then repeat the process. Do the same with the other foot.

- Now move to one of your legs. Stretch it out as far as you can and really feel the tension from your thighs to your calves. And then to your bottom. Let go and repeat the process. Do the same with the other leg.

- Think about one of your hands next. Tighten your hand into a fist. Feel the tightness in your fingers. Repeat and do the exercise again with the other hand.

- Next your arms. In turn stretch out one arm, then the other, and then let go and feel your arms relax as they return to their original position and become limp and floppy.

- Now become aware of your tummy. Really tense and pull in your stomach muscles. Then push the muscles outwards. Relax and repeat the process.

- Your back now. Arch it, hold and relax. Do this twice.

- Pull your shoulders back as you tighten them. Release and repeat. Lift your shoulders to your ears and let go. Repeat.

- Now think about your face. Start by tightening and then relaxing the muscles in your forehead and around your eyes. Frown and then let go. Move on to the muscles around your mouth and jaws. Push your lips tightly together and clench your teeth. Really feel the tension before you let it go and repeat the exercise.

- Push your tongue firmly first to the roof and then to the floor of your mouth. Do this twice, relaxing it between each push.

- Before you finish your practice, take a moment to notice your body and how it feels. Notice the relaxation there and how you feel. Take your time to get up again. You may want to stretch out your body to return it to normal.

Routledge
Taylor & Francis Group

Techniques for head and neck relaxation

- Sit or stand in a comfortable position.
- Drop your head forward towards your chest and then slowly pull it back to a central position as you notice the muscles in the back of your neck.
- Drop your head to one side towards the shoulder and notice the muscle movement. Repeat this movement on the other side.
- Drop your head down and roll it gently to one side, back to the centre and then to the other side. Repeat several times.

Techniques for facial relaxation

- Rub your cheeks, jaw and forehead and then let go of any tension.
- Raise your eyebrows and then relax them. Repeat, but this time frown.
- Clench your teeth and then relax your jaws.
- Stick your tongue out as far as it will go, then pull it back and let it rest gently in your mouth.
- Push your lips forward as if you are blowing an exaggerated kiss and then pull them back as if you are making an exaggerated smile. Relax.
- Pretend to chew some sticky toffee for several seconds.
- Do a big yawn.

Routledge

11 | Breathing

The perceived association between breathing difficulties and stammering has been apparent in the literature since the beginning of the last century. Breathing is also frequently reported by many clients as an area of difficulty and one which they feel has a direct link with their stammering. Despite numerous studies it remains unclear, however, whether disruptions in normal breathing are a by-product of stammering or indeed an explanation in themselves. Since the last edition of this book there has been no evidence that would contradict the view we then held: that it seems unlikely to be the latter.

However, many clinicians, including ourselves, still feel it is important to explain the mechanics of breathing to clients (see Chapter 5 'Identification' and the normal speech production questionnaire in Chapter 3) along with other aspects of speech production. Understanding the mechanics of normal speech production helps a client to know what he is aiming for and the areas he may need to work at to achieve his goal.

In line with speech therapy programmes for other client groups, the basic aims of respiration therapy are for the client to:

- have a basic knowledge of the mechanisms needed for breathing, and especially breathing for speech
- establish good breathing patterns using the intercostal muscles and the diaphragm
- develop good lung capacity
- learn to control inhalation and exhalation, and coordinate the muscles involved.

When to use

Breathing work is often carried out after preliminary work on relaxation. Where breathing is to be worked on in isolation, then residual tension may play a part. Mathieson (2001) suggests that posture is also checked before work begins on breathing. Particular aspects to look out for include round shoulders and a general sagging posture. The position of the head is also important: it should be held in alignment with the spinal column (see Handout 9 'Good posture' in Chapter 2). Most clinicians recommend that work on breathing should be carried out when the client and clinician are standing, preferably in front of a mirror. The client should be encouraged to observe his breathing pattern in the mirror rather than look down at his diaphragm.

Indications for working on breathing might be when clients present with any of the following:

• speaking when running out of air

• lack of time taken to breathe

• lack of coordination between respiration and phonation

• evidence of speaking on an ingressive airstream

• over-frequent inhalation, possibly leading on occasions to hyperventilation

• not taking in enough air

• gasping for air

• letting air out too quickly.

How to teach good breathing

We find it helpful to introduce two main concepts: capacity and control. Both are essential for good breathing. Some clients may have problems in both areas; others may have good capacity but poor control over exhalation. The exercises selected will therefore be dependent on good initial identification in both areas. In addition, a client may need to work on coordination of breathing and phonation. Below we list activities for all three areas. In addition to these exercises, a client may need to pay attention to two points:

1   The frequency of his breathing: if breathing is too frequent it may produce symptoms of hyperventilation or make speech sound disjointed. If breathing is too infrequent, the voice may become strained.

2   The time taken for each breath: more time given to breathing can produce a more relaxed feeling to speech; rushed breathing can increase tension.

In order for work on breathing to be effective and for changed breathing patterns to become established, a client needs to commit to practising at home what he has learned in the clinic. Without this, the strong habit factor of poor breathing patterns is likely to preclude any lasting change.

Common problems

• There is an argument that the introduction of breathing exercises may be counter-productive as it can result in an increase in tension. However, most clinicians agree that where 'speech breathing patterns are affected by anxiety and tension, the problem is compounded by the compensatory strategies that may subsequently evolve… As a result, patients may need information and practice in appropriate speech breathing patterns' (Mathieson, 2001, p64).

• Martin & Lockhart note that 'breathing exercises can produce unexpected and uncomfortable emotional responses in patients' (2000, p119). They advise that this is usually a normal reaction and one that clinicians can usually deal with by offering the person time to recover and talk. On some occasions, however, they suggest that an onward expert referral may be warranted.

We have listed other possible problems under the specific activities to which they refer.

Activities for breathing

Checking breathing patterns ⓘ ⚙

Before starting work on breathing, it is helpful for the client to have an indication of the type of breathing he typically uses. For this exercise the client is instructed to place one hand on his chest and the other on his abdomen. He then breathes in. He is asked in which hand he notices movement first. If it is his lower hand he is breathing abdominally. If, however, it is his upper hand which moves, his breathing is likely to be clavicular.

Encouraging diaphragmatic breathing – lying down ⓘ

A client may find it very difficult to grasp the concept of diaphragmatic breathing. If this is the case he can be helped by asking him to lie on the floor with a reasonably heavy book on his abdomen. He then aims to use his abdominal muscles to make the book move up and down. Once he can feel where the movement should be, he can repeat the exercise with one hand pressed down on the abdomen instead of the book. Once he is confident about the movement he is aiming for, he can then move on to the other exercises described below.

Encouraging diaphragmatic breathing – standing up ⓘ

Clinician and client stand up facing a mirror. The clinician demonstrates to the client where he should position his hands to feel diaphragmatic movement and correct movement of his intercostal muscles. This can be with one hand over the diaphragm, on the abdominal wall just above waist level, and the other placed against the lower ribs on one side. Alternatively, the client can place his hands flat on his ribs with fingers meeting at the breastbone.

The client is instructed to breathe in once through the nose and gently out through the mouth, while monitoring muscle and ribcage movement. Specific attention may be drawn to general clavicular tension and/or clavicular movement during inhalation as appropriate. In order to avoid hyperventilation the clinician should not allow the client to repeat this exercise without a pause or rest in between attempts.

Common problems

Clinicians should be on the lookout for a number of difficulties that may arise out of the previous task. Careful monitoring by the clinician will be necessary initially, but as time goes on the client should be more able to self-correct.

- The client may take in an excessive volume of air, possibly because he recalls the 'stop, take a deep breath' instructions that he may have heard as a child.

- The client may increase his tension levels in an attempt to perform the task 'to the best of his abilities'.

- The client may respond with 'reverse breathing', that is, pulling the abdomen in when asked to breathe in and pushing it out on breathing out. This is a common problem. We find it is helpful for the client to think in terms of 'breathe in = movement out', 'breathe out = movement in'. Once the client equates the concept of breathing in with making internal space, this problem is usually solved.

- Inspiration may be noisy due to tension in the larynx.

- Posture may deteriorate as the exercise progresses.

There are one or two clients in our experience who have found these first exercises particularly difficult. On these occasions we have worked on relaxation techniques and returned to the breathing work at a later stage, once general relaxation can be achieved.

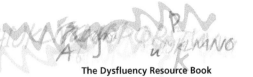
Extending exhalation time ⓘ

This exercise helps a client to develop control over his breathing. The clinician should first demonstrate normal quick inhalation followed by a prolonged exhalation as required for speech. Martin & Lockhart (2000) suggest inspiration to a count of three and gradually increasing expiration in stages to an eventual count of six or however many feels comfortable for each individual. Concentrating more on the exhalation than the inhalation phase will help to reduce any build-up of tension in the upper chest or any tendency to hyperventilate.

Following this, the client can increase the length of the phrase he speaks. Mathieson (2001) suggests he uses a phrase such as, 'One is all I need; one, two is all I need; one, two, three is all I need'. The client continues increasing the length of the phrase in this way until full capacity has been reached, but without using reserve or residual air. Another suggestion of Mathieson's is that the client builds up a phrase in the following way: 'It was a cold day. It was a cold and windy day. It was a cold, windy and wet day', and so on (2001, p508).

Common problems

• Breath escapes between each count.

• The ribs are held in an elevated position during counting and then lowered as the client reaches the end of the breath or the end of the counting.

Extending exhalation time for speech ⓘ

In our clinical experience a number of adult clients have had significantly reduced exhalation for speech. We have assumed that this was due to poor breathing patterns and, indeed, this appears to have been borne out by subsequent improvement following breathing exercises. These recommendations are therefore made to clinicians:

1 Obtain a baseline measure, such as the number of seconds a client can sustain production of a single vowel, at the outset of work on respiration.

2 Once a baseline is calculated, work can begin on the production of a number of voiceless fricatives (such as 's', 'sh' and 'f'), achieving a recommended duration of approximately 20 seconds (in a healthy, fit male client).

3 Having reached this consistently, the client should then be encouraged to move on to vowel sounds.

In this way the client can concentrate on breathing for speech before having to focus on coordination, exhalation and phonation. It is useful to draw the client's attention to the quality of the sound he is working on, encouraging him to listen and try to maintain even pitch, tone and loudness levels. Martin & Lockhart (2000) stress that the client should always be aiming for good *quality* of sound in his practice. *Quantity* is less important.

Coordination of exhalation and phonation ⓘ

In addition to work on capacity and control, some clients will benefit from work to help them coordinate their breathing and voice production. The following principles apply to these exercises:

• Attention should be given to beginning phonation as soon after inhalation as possible (Boone *et al*, 2005). Thus, the client is not wasting a lot of the outgoing air before phonation starts and then running out of air prematurely as a result.

• The client imitates the clinician's modelling of quick oral inhalation and slow expiration (Mathieson, 2001). This is repeated with the client counting slowly, first to 6 and then gradually increasing up to 20, all following the rapid inhalation.

• The client is encouraged to gradually increase the length of utterance produced on one exhalation, working from an easy sigh to phrases of five words (Bonnard, 1996). The following exercise is an example:

1 Yawn and give a gentle sigh as you breathe out.

2 Breathe in, then out, saying:

he

how

har

hoe

hoo

3 Say the following words on a sigh as you breathe out:

hat

him

hit

hill

house

home

hum

hymn

hat

hutch

his

horn

4 Say the following words on an easy outward breath:

much

more

many

men

mean

male

mink

mint

5 Then combine two together:

much more

many men

Mike meant

my mill

6   Try other combinations on one breath:

meal time

milk van

main street

melting ice

meek and mild

make a meal

marrying kind

moaning mother

many more boys

meaningful day

7   Finally, some longer phrases to attempt:

main meal of the morning

Mike is more mean than you

don't make a meal of it

maybe there isn't much more

mountain men search far and wide.

The sentences in the easy onset exercise in Chapter 13 (p175) can also be used for breathing practice.

Handout ⓘ ⚙

Handouts 40 and 41 can be used as a basis for the breathing exercises detailed above.

Breathing exercises: a 10-point programme

1 When you breathe in, you need to make space in your lungs for the air you are taking in. Efficient breathing involves the movement of the diaphragm and intercostal (between the ribs) muscles to make the space available for the incoming air. When you breathe out, you use the same muscles to ensure the air is expelled from your lungs again.

2 Place your hand at the bottom of your ribcage. Take an easy breath in through your nose and out through your mouth. You should feel your diaphragm move down and out and your ribcage move up and out.

3 When you breathe out, let the air out slowly and gently. You should feel your diaphragm move up and in and your ribcage move down and in.

4 Take some slow, long breaths. Breathe in through your nose for a count of three seconds and then out through your mouth, also for a count of three. This should feel relaxing. Pause briefly after each attempt. Stop if at any time you feel dizzy or lightheaded (this can indicate that you are 'over-breathing').

5 Now as you breathe out, let out a sigh.

6 Gradually extend the length of the sigh, but keep that relaxed feeling. Do not push the last bit of air out or push the sigh out.

7 Now as you breathe out, try letting the air escape in short stages or puffs until you feel you have got rid of all of your air. Do not top up the air with another breath in between.

8 When we speak, we are breathing out. Try this last exercise again, this time saying the sound 'sh'. As you breathe out, try saying this sound gently.

9 This time break down the sound into chunks: 'sh, sh, sh'. Remember to use just one outward breath.

10 Try making the 'sh' sound, first quietly, then louder, then finally quietly again.

Remember: adopt an upright posture, preferably standing in front of a mirror. Keep your shoulders still and lowered. Keep as relaxed as possible. Stop between each exercise and stop immediately if you feel dizzy.

Routledge
Taylor & Francis Group

Good breathing

In order to breathe well you need to have a relaxed and comfortable posture.

• You should keep upright, but your spine should not be rigid or tense.

• Your head needs to be facing forwards.

• Your shoulders should be relaxed and not hunched or rounded.

Diaphragmatic breathing

This is the most efficient and least effortful sort of breathing. As the name implies, it uses your diaphragm, which is a dome-shaped muscle in your abdomen, below your lungs. The intercostal muscles (the ones between your ribs) are also involved. There should be little movement in your shoulders and upper chest when you breathe. It helps to breathe in through your nose (the air gets warmed up in that way and this helps it to move through your body more freely). Breathe out through your mouth – this is what we do when we speak.

When you breathe in:

• the diaphragm contracts and moves downwards and outwards

• the ribs move upwards and outwards

• your chest gets bigger as your lungs fill with air.

When you breathe out:

• the diaphragm relaxes and moves upwards and inwards

• the ribs move downwards and inwards

• the air leaves your lungs and your chest gets smaller again.

Routledge

12 | Rate control

In the past, work on a client's rate of speech has meant imposing a consistently slow pace across all his utterances. Techniques such as slow speech, a method popular in the 1970s, taught clients to regulate their speech to a prescribed number of syllables or words per minute and, using a behavioural approach, structured speech into units of increasing length and/ or complexity. For example, the *Monterey Fluency Program* (used mainly with children) used sentences of increasing length and gradually extended the amount of speaking time required from the client (Ryan & Van Kirk, 1971).

Our thinking in this area has developed considerably since then. We no longer promote the use of a consistent rate across all speech, nor do we teach rate control rigidly in terms of syllables per minute. Now rate is viewed as a more dynamic unit that a speaker will adjust and change according to his circumstances.

When to use

Rate control is a fluency-enhancing technique suitable for clients:

- who, in conversation, try to match the speaking rate of other people, which may adversely affect their own fluency

- who have no strategies to slow down their rate

- whose fluency is disrupted by a faster rate of speech

- who may report a generally fast life style, that is, they walk fast, eat quickly, and their speech is a further extension of this pattern.

Rate control should usually be taught after identification, desensitisation and avoidance reduction. It may also be taught alongside other fluency-controlling techniques such as easy onset and good breathing.

Teaching rate control

Before embarking on changing the speed of a client's speech, we may ask him to experiment with changing the rate of an activity unrelated to speech (see Chapter 4 'Variation: non-speech and speech'). For example, we may ask him to change the speed at which he:

- showers or washes in the morning

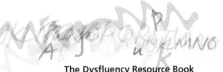

- cleans his teeth

- eats his lunch

- uses the computer

- walks to his house or flat

- takes off his coat or jacket

- reads a newspaper or book (silently to himself).

This will help the client engage in a change process and may loosen any notion he has that activities have to be carried out at a certain pace. It can also illustrate to him how slowing down is quite difficult to achieve because we all have certain patterns of behaviour we perform without thought or attention.

In teaching rate control we ask an adult who stammers to consider the speed of his speech in the context of the communication situation. He is asked to identify the variables that may affect his rate. A typical list would include:

- the content of the utterance

- the context

- the listener

- the speaker's mood, affect and physical state, for example, level of tiredness

- the speaker's confidence level in the situation

- the speaker's perceived need for control and/or fluency.

The analogy of driving a car and modifying the speed of the car according to the road conditions, driver's well-being, engine capacity, and so on, is useful to apply to teaching a client the value of a flexible approach to rate control. Webster & Poulos use the same analogy, applying it to speech targets generally:

> Adapting your target use to speaking situations is like shifting gears in a car. If the road is bad, you shift to a lower gear to give yourself better control. When the car is moving more slowly you can better monitor and control its movement and have time to prepare for difficulties. If you always drive in high gear, ignoring the condition of the road surface and other traffic around you, at some point you will lose control.
> Speech is no different.
> (1989, p67)

This notion of flexibility is promoted in the choice of methods presented to a client. Rather than advocate a single way of achieving a slower rate (for example, in the slowed speech technique of the 1970s, the decrease in rate is achieved by lengthening or extending all articulatory contacts), we illustrate that a slower speed of speech can be attained in a number of ways. These are summarised as:

- increased pausing, in line with phrase and sentence boundaries

- increasing the duration of the vowel or the length of time the articulators are in contact with each other

- increasing the length of time taken to breathe.

Let us consider each of these in turn.

Pausing

It is important that the client is aware of the significance of gaps or silences in his speech. Too often, he is acutely aware of breaks in his speech and associates them with dysfluency. He needs to be reminded of other possible reasons for pausing, for example:

- to think
- to breathe
- to attend to the context and the needs of listeners
- to emphasise a word or a point of view
- to gain greater control over emotions.

(Readers may like to use Handout 42 'Why should I pause?' to discuss these points in more detail with individuals or groups of clients.)

A client is encouraged to experiment with pausing either at the beginning of his utterance, that is, before he speaks, or to use pauses where he would use punctuation such as full stops or commas in written language. In this way the pause correlates with the meaning of what he is saying.

Changes in speech production

In terms of speech production, the generally accepted way of reducing rate is to slow down the articulatory movements. This results in prolonged contact of the articulators during, for example, production of fricatives, affricates and nasals. Vowels and semi-vowels and/or continuants require a lengthening of production; however, plosives are more problematic. It is recommended that the stop phase of a plosive is not unduly maintained as this could precipitate a block due to the excess build-up of intra-oral air pressure. An alternative is to reduce the stop phase so that the production of the plosive sounds more like a fricative.

In general, it is easier to prolong vowels than consonants. This tends to create an even stress pattern, not unlike that produced by the use of syllable-timed speech. It can be difficult to eliminate this later in therapy and the resulting speech can sound 'different' to listeners and often to the clients themselves. A more natural pattern can be achieved if a client prolongs both consonants and vowels from the outset. More acceptable intonation configurations may be worked on later.

It is especially important to prolong the initial phoneme of an utterance and/or breath group as this is most often dysfluent. We suggest to a client that he eases or slides into his first word and then says the rest of the sentence normally.

Breathing

There is a separate chapter on breathing (Chapter 11), but we have also included breathing here as there are important issues in relation to rate control. The crucial point for a client is the time it takes to breathe. As previously stated, a person who stammers can equate silence with blocking and needs to be encouraged to develop a tolerance to the silence that ensues during an in-breath.

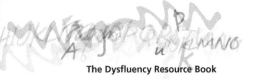
Common problems

These can be summarised as follows:

• The client generally has a fast pace of life, making change difficult.

• The client is unable to tolerate silence.

• He experiences feelings of urgency.

• He is anxious about losing his speaking turn in a conversation or discussion.

Activities for rate control

Practising pausing

The client is given Handout 42 'Why should I pause?' and encouraged to experiment with pausing in the following activities.

Sentences 🛈 ⚙

The client uses a pause to give emphasis to different words in these sentences. Vary where the pause comes to give different emphasis.

Single sentences

A rolling stone gathers no moss.

There are green and yellow curtains at the back of it.

You and I both know that the truth is altogether something different.

I prefer the one I saw you with last weekend in Leeds.

Have you any idea how much time it takes to make one of those?

I am going out and I don't think I shall be back in time to walk the dog.

I don't think that it is any use trying to reach him by phone at this time of day.

Actually I think it will rain today despite what the weatherman said.

You should go and see the doctor and get checked out before you go into work.

If you carry on like this I think there is a possibility that you will do yourself an injury.

I would like you to sit down for a minute and listen to what I have to say.

All this time and effort will surely pay off for you in the end.

Two sentences

The best film I ever saw was one I never expected to like. It was not even one that I would have chosen to see.

My favourite restaurant is in the south of the country on the lakeside. They serve fresh fish straight out of the lake and cook it in front of you.

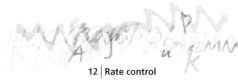

I went to the football match yesterday with all the guys from work. Our team was winning but there was an equaliser in the last minute and the final score was a draw.

He went into town to get the music he had heard the band play the night before. Unfortunately, the shop was not open because it was early closing that day.

The children were badly behaved because there was nothing for them to play with. Usually they are very good and will sit for hours playing computer games or watching TV.

By making simple changes to your life regular exercise can become part of your daily routine. You could swim before breakfast, bike to work, run up the stairs and go for a jog at lunchtime!

Reading a short paragraph

A client is asked to read out a short passage from a newspaper or book. His attention is drawn to the punctuation (commas, full stops and so on) as a way of cueing him into using pauses. The clinician may suggest that he counts one second for a comma, two for a full stop and so on to encourage a long enough pause initially.

The following is an example of a useful passage (with plenty of punctuation!).

> Deep down here by the dark water lived old Gollum, a small slimy creature. I don't know where he came from, nor who or what he was. He was Gollum – as dark as darkness, except for two big round pale eyes in his thin face. He had a little boat, and he rowed about quite quietly on the lake; for lake it was, wide and deep and deadly cold. He paddled it with large feet dangling over the side, but never a ripple did he make. Not he. He was looking out of his pale lamp-like eyes for blind fish, which he grabbed with his long fingers as quick as thinking. He liked meat too. Goblin he thought good, when he could get it; but he took care they never found him out. He just throttled them from behind, if they ever came down alone anywhere near the edge of the water, while he was prowling about. They very seldom did, for they had a feeling that something unpleasant was lurking down there, down at the very roots of the mountain.
> (From *The Hobbit* by JRR Tolkien)

Practising different ways of controlling rate

Handout ⓘ ⚙

Using Handout 43 'Ways to change the speed of your speech', discuss with the client ways of experimenting with each of the methods described. Reading is a good way to start experimentation. However, it is recommended that the client moves from reading practice to more spontaneous speech work as soon as possible.

Short monologues ⓘ ⚙

A client can use this activity to practise pausing, making sure he pauses before he begins to speak and at regular intervals while speaking. (When working with groups, other clients can be encouraged to remind the person speaking to pause if he becomes too involved in the content of his speech and forgets to do this.) In addition, the client should be encouraged to try to control his rate by either changing his speech production (that is, extending articulatory contacts) or taking a longer time to breathe.

With these issues in mind, ask the client to describe the following:

• how to lose weight

- how to iron a shirt

- how to investigate a murder

- how to decorate a Christmas tree

- how to make friends with a member of the opposite sex

- how to make spaghetti bolognese

- how to move house

- how to choose a holiday

- how to stop smoking

- how to rob a bank.

Questions and answers ⓘ ⚙

Further practice on experimentation with ways of controlling rate can be carried out on more interactive speech tasks. One option is a question and answer based task. This can be organised in group therapy as a 'Mastermind' type activity or in individual therapy as a '20 questions' game. Another option is to have group members ask each other questions on selected topics which have not been predetermined (they can be written on cards which are placed in a pile in front of the client/s). Some themes for questions are:

- naming characters from TV programmes

- place names/capitals

- famous people's names

- identifying flags

- identifying singers or bands who sang named songs

- naming the ingredients of main dishes and desserts, such as lasagne, sherry trifle

- 'Who said?': identifying the originators of famous quotations or sayings.

Presentations ⓘ ⚙

Each client prepares a 3–5-minute talk on a given topic. Presentations are given in a formal manner, with a client standing and using visual aids as appropriate. Video recording is also recommended here. On completion of the talk, the individual is given immediate feedback on the rate control method he has used. The topic may be suggested by group members, or, in the case of individual therapy, may be supplied. Here are some suggestions:

- If I ruled the world

- Winning the lottery

- How I spend my leisure time

- A favourite holiday

- A family story

- My early childhood

- If I could build my own house …

'People in houses' ⓘ ⚙

Pre-printed postcards are given to group members. Each client has a couple of minutes' thinking time, after which he reads out the name and address on his card to the whole group or clinicians. He is then required to describe the person on the card in as much detail as he can. Aspects of appearance, residence, occupation, personality, life style and so on can be included. The following are examples of names and addresses:

Colonel C.J. Stonebrow-Smythe DSO
Officers' Mess
The Barracks
Carrick Camp
Carrick
Yorkshire

Mr George Snodgrass
3 Railway Cuttings
Wolverhampton

Miss Emily Jane Littlelove
Rose Cottage
Leafy Hollow Lane
Wold-on-the-Water
Hertfordshire

Rev. Jonathan Humble
The Vicarage
Lower Chivington
Nr Winchester

Mr & Mrs Fred Jackson
Bon Accord
Seaview Court
Weston-super-Mare

Dr Roselea Clara Hughes MA, RCM
Flat 2 Ground Floor
Mary Pickles House
University Court
Cambridge

Hamish MacTavish
The Keeper's Croft
Ross Estate
Loch Ross
Nr Tarbot
Scotland

Ms George Greenlea
Tutor's Lodge
Blue House
Ribbon Preparatory School for Young Ladies
Hanging Haversham
Nr Arundel

Miss Susan C. Quinn
The Dance & Ballroom Centre
10 Fox Trot Court
Cheltenham
Gloucestershire

Farmer John Giles
The Barn
Stony Lane
Lower Bottom
Alwoodley
Accrington

Why should I pause?

Here are some reasons why you should pause:

Thinking time

- To work out what to say (ie sorting out your ideas, opinions)
- To work out how to say what you have decided to say (ie putting your ideas into a sentence structure)
- To select the appropriate vocabulary, retrieving it from the 'dictionary' in your head

Breathing

- You need time to regularly take in air

Breathing usually occurs at the beginning of a sentence or phrase and also during 'ums' and 'ers' (in normal fluent speakers). How many words anyone can speak in one breath varies from person to person. On average a breath for speech will last three or four seconds, but can be 'stretched' to 12 seconds. The amount of air you take in on one breath will depend on what you think you are going to say. If you anticipate a longer sentence you will automatically take in more air.

Listeners' needs

- To check that the listener(s) has taken in or is taking in the content of what you are saying
- To allow the listener(s) time to assimilate or interject and ask for clarification if necessary
- To make what you are saying sound more interesting for your listener

Emphasis

- To add weight or emphasis to what you are saying

Emotions

- To give you time to control your emotions when something you are saying is upsetting, makes you angry, excited or agitated in some other way
- To make your emotions clear, if this is what you choose to do

Urgency factor

- To reduce the feelings of urgency

You may experience these feelings before or after stammering. In these instances an increased speed of speech is used either to get through a stammer or to 'get away' from it as quickly as possible after it has occurred. Sometimes individuals have a generally fast speed of speech, as if talking is an unpleasant activity which must be hurried through to get it over with. Alternatively, speed of speech can be associated with fluency and you may find that you talk more rapidly during fluent periods, thinking that this 'cannot last and I'm sure to stammer in a minute'.

Routledge

Ways to change the speed of your speech

1 Increase the number of pauses

- Pause before speaking

- Pause when you might put a comma or a full stop in your speech
  (if it were written down)

2 Take time to compose your sentences

- Think of interesting ways of saying what you have to say

- Insert an interesting word or two into your speech

- Don't talk 'round the houses'. Be concise where you can

3 Don't rush into speaking

- Pretend to think

- Count to three

- Consider your response if you are answering a question

4 Take time to breathe

- Breathe at the beginning of your utterance

- If you have lots to say, breathe at 'meaningful points', such as the end of a phrase or sentence

5 Stretch the sounds of your speech slightly

- At the beginning of an utterance try sliding into the first sound of the first word

6 Use a slower speed when saying a word on which you anticipate having difficulty

- Relax your speech muscles before saying it

- 'Go into it' more slowly

- Extend the slower pace through the word; don't rush through it

7 Consider your listener

- Give them time to take in what you are saying

- Give them the opportunity to ask a question. It will help them to understand or clarify what you are telling them

8 Speed up your speech

- When you know what you are going to say

- When you feel more confident

- When you are comfortable with the other people around you

- When your speech is more fluent

Routledge
Taylor & Francis Group

13 | Easy onset

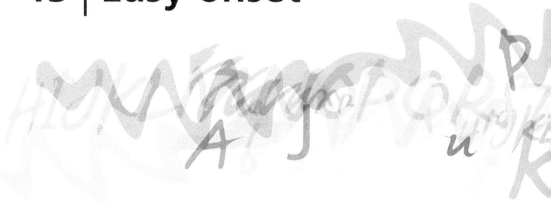

Easy onset is a fluency technique that was developed following research on laryngeal function. The results of a number of studies seemed to suggest that some adults who stammered had difficulty coordinating respiration and phonation when initiating speech. Proving popular in programmes in the 1970s in the USA (Webster, 1974; Cooper, 1979), this technique provided a means to address this issue. When carrying out an easy onset, the individual is encouraged to start an utterance with a small amount of exhaled air, then the sound of the first word follows in an easy manner. Thus the speaker breaks down the start of speech into its constituent parts, rather than attempting to simultaneously coordinate respiration, voice production and articulation.

When to use

Easy onset is an excellent technique for clients who:

- have disrupted breathing patterns
- have silent or audible blocks at the beginning of an utterance
- stammer primarily at the beginning of a breath group
- have tense articulation and/or hard vocal attack.

Teaching easy onsets

Teaching easy onsets should follow any therapy that is needed on breathing, relaxation, posture and light articulatory contacts, as these are prerequisites for the technique. The technique can be summarised as follows:

1 relaxed posture, including upper chest, neck and articulators

2 correct (diaphragmatic) breathing pattern; the client should be able to use quick inhalation and extended exhalation (see Chapter 11 'Breathing')

3 light articulatory contacts.

Once these features have been established the client should be instructed to:

(a) take in a normal relaxed breath

(b) exhale a small amount of air

(c) begin to say the first sound of the word or utterance

(d) while saying this sound, slightly extend the length of the articulatory contact.

Note For plosive sounds the client should be encouraged to shorten the stop phase and prolong the release stage.

Clinical practice

Stage 1
Practice should be carried out first on single phonemes. A recommended order is:

1 vowels

2 approximants/continuants/liquids

3 nasals

4 fricatives and affricates

5 plosives.

Stage 2
The client produces words of increasing length and complexity. Start with simple monosyllabic words, both nonsense and meaningful (CV, CVC), and move up to the most complex structures (CCCVCCC) and polysyllabic words. (For simple monosyllabic nonsense and meaningful words see Activity 2 below.) Then finally move on to phrases and simple sentences (see Activity 3).

Stage 3
Once the technique can be produced on request (at random) in reading, then the clinician may introduce spontaneous speech exercises, for example:

• question and answer tasks, requiring a single word answer, followed by

• a two-word response

• a short phrase (see Activity 5)

• monologues (see Activity 6)

• picture descriptions

• conversational and discussion work (see Activity 7).

In the initial stages of reading, monologue and conversation, the clinician should indicate where the client should use the easy onset technique. In later stages this is phased out and the client takes increasing responsibility for deciding where he needs to use it (that is, when he is experiencing difficulty and/or anticipating difficulty).

A further description of the establishment and development of the easy onset technique can be found in Stewart & Turnbull (2007) and a summary is shown in Table 13.1.

Common problems

Problems that indicate tension

- There is clavicular or other associated movement during breathing and/or phonation.
- The exhalation phase sounds like a 'h' (there may be diaphragmatic tension or tension at the laryngeal level).
- The client blows out air in a forceful manner rather than letting a small amount out (diaphragmatic tension).
- The client exhales a small amount of air, then stops the air flow before saying the first sound (laryngeal and/or articulatory tension).
- There is vocal cord closure (laryngeal tension).
- The client produces a rising inflection as phonation is initiated (laryngeal tension).

Problems requiring further work on breathing pattern

- There is clavicular tension.
- Inspiration time is too long.
- The client is letting out too much exhaled air.
- The client blows exhaled air out in a forceful manner.
- The client exhales a small amount of air, then stops the air flow before initiating phonation.

Other problems

- The client is able to start phonation but then stammers on the phoneme. This is often due to lack of soft articulatory contacts and/or specific tension in the oral muscles or articulators themselves.
- The client prolongs the vowel or other following phoneme, instead of, or in addition to, the first sound. (In extreme cases a client may slow his production of all the sounds in the word, not just the initial one.) This is not a major problem but it affects the degree of naturalness that can be achieved and the technique may be quite noticeable to the listener in the long term.

Table 13.1 Exercise for practising easy onset at different levels of difficulty

Single phoneme	Word level	Phrase level	Sentence level
/aː/ or 'ah'	art	art for art's sake	Art galleries should remain free and open for everyone to enjoy our heritage
/ɑ/	at	at the same time	At the same time I can see your point of view
/i/ or 'ee'	even	even I know that	Evening can be the best part of the day
/ɪ/	it	it isn't the same	It isn't the same as the last time we were here
/ɒ/	orange	oranges are good	Oranges are grown in the sunny state of Florida
/ʌ/	umbrella	umbrellas for sale	Umbrellas come in a variety of sizes and colours
/w/	where	where are you?	Where are you going with my car keys?
/h/	how	how many?	How many times do I have to say it?
/l/	look	look at this	Look at this set of photos I have just had developed
/y/	you	you are kind	You are kind to me when I need help
/r/	read	read the paper	Read the paper, now try this book
/f/	fish	fish and chips	Fish and chips is my favourite meal
/v/	very	very many people	Very many people go to the coast on a bank holiday
/θ/	think	thinking time	Thinking time is what I need most
/ð/	those	those people	Those people over there have just moved into our street
/s/	sowing	sowing seeds	Sowing seeds in my greenhouse gives me a lot of pleasure
/z/	zoo	zoo animals	Zoo animals should be kept in better conditions
/ʃ/ or 'sh'	sugar	sugar and spice	Sugar and spices are often sold at the delicatessen shop in the high street
/tʃ/ or 'sh'	chop	chopsticks from China	Chopsticks from China are tricky to use with some foods
/dʒ/ or 'j'	judges	judges in court	Judges appear in courts throughout the country
/p/	please	please can I?	Please can I have that one over there?
/b/	before	before he left	Before he left he changed everything around
/t/	to	to be or not to be	'To be or not to be, that is the question'

Single phoneme	Word level	Phrase level	Sentence level
/d/	don't	don't leave it	Don't leave it too long before you call again
/k/	Katy	Katy's bag	Katy's bag was left in the library on Friday
/g/	go	go to the left	Go to the left and it is the first door facing you

Activities

Activity 1 Easy onset at sound level ⓘ

The client is asked to produce specific sounds from particular categories (refer to the section on normal speech production in Chapter 3), for example, all sounds produced by the narrowing of articulators (fricatives), all sounds produced by a build-up of air pressure behind articulators (plosives). The clinician may model each sound prior to the client's production and then phase her model out, allowing the client to produce each sound on presentation of a visual cue only.

Activity 2 Easy onset at monosyllabic level ⓘ

Using Handout 44 'Practising easy onset at monosyllabic word level', the client is asked to produce simple monosyllabic words and nonsense words. The phoneme in the centre can be changed as the client practises different groups of sounds. Similarly, different vowels and diphthongs in the outside boxes may be used to vary the exercise.

Activity 3 Easy onset at sentence level ⓘ

The client is asked to complete the following sentences with a two-word (minimum) phrase.

Please go and buy me ....

The best thing to eat is..

The greatest invention is ....

My earliest memory is ....

I'd love to visit ....

My mother/father always used to ....

Television today is ....

If it rains at the weekend I..

Children are really good at ....

As a child I used to ....

If I were a politician I would ....

When I have spare time I usually ....

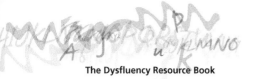

People who go to work on their bicycle are ....

I know some people run marathons but I...

Having a brother/sister should be ....

Music when I was younger was ....

Playing a musical instrument is often ....

Celebrities who appear on red carpets always ....

Drinking coffee first thing in the morning ....

On Sundays I always like to ....

Activity 4 Random reading ⓘ

The clinician marks every tenth word in a reading passage. The client is asked to read and carry out an easy onset on the first sound of the marked words.

Activity 5 Asking questions ⓘ

The client and clinician take turns in asking each other questions such as the following:

One-word level

What is your favourite food?

What is your favourite colour?

What number house do you live in?

How many letters are in your first name?

How long did it take you to get here today?

Which is your favourite city to visit?

Two-word level

What car do you drive and what colour is it?

Tell me the name of your favourite film star/actor/actress?

How long have you lived in your current house?

What alliterative adjective goes with your name, for example, troublesome Trudy, joyful Jackie?

If you woke up one day and had to choose to spend a day as a US president or a Buddist monk, which would you choose?

Variation for groups

In a group context, individuals can make up questions to ask other group members. Feedback should be given on the quality of the easy onset at the beginning of each answer.

Activity 6 Speaking ⓘ ⚙

A client is asked to speak for an allotted time period (for example, one or two minutes) on a topic from the list below, or, if in a group, on a topic provided by a group member.

Monologue topics

Learning to drive a car

Doing DIY

Gardening in the spring

Stargazing

Cooking for friends

Going on a picnic

Holidays in Britain

Childhood friends

Moving house/flat

Starting school

Activity 7 Conversation and discussion ⓘ ⚙

The following topics can be used in both individual and group sessions. Clients should be encouraged to set specific easy onset 'targets' to be achieved in the course of the conversation.

Conversation or discussion topics

Parents should teach their children to drive

Television should be more educational

Would you say you lived a 'green' life style?

Our society is more accepting of violence than it was in the past

Football players are paid too much money

The Royal Family does much to promote Britain abroad

Teenagers should be introduced to voluntary work in the community before leaving school

Local produce could be sold more cheaply by supermarkets

What do you think about the nutritional advice given to the public, for example, eat five fruits and vegetables per day?

All children should be able to speak more than one language

Practising easy onset at monosyllabic word level

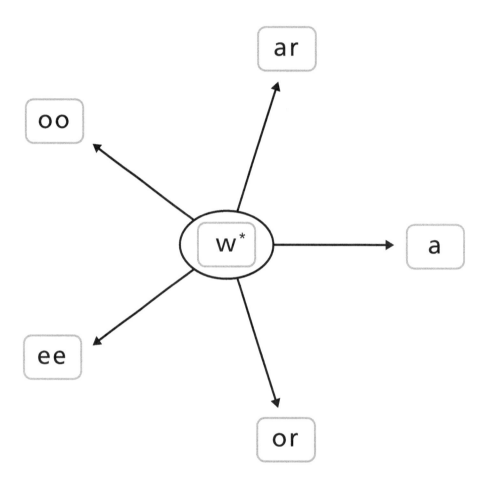

* Insert different phonemes in centre to develop client's proficiency

Routledge
Taylor & Francis Group

14 | Block modification

For most clinicians the words 'block modification' are immediately associated with the name Van Riper (1973, 1982). These techniques come from his work of 20 years, investigating the speech of very severe stammerers and experimenting with a variety of therapeutic approaches. The aim of block modification was not to train people to be fluent, but rather to stutter 'fluently'. Van Riper's premise was that the core of stammering is probably what he refers to as 'lags and mistimings', which are neuromuscular in origin. He saw the associated struggle and avoidance, however, as learned behaviours which can be unlearned (Van Riper, 1990). These behaviours are what perpetuate the stammer as a disabling disorder and, if they can be modified, Van Riper proposes that most of the problem will no longer exist. From his studies, Van Riper came to believe that as a person anticipates stammering, they 'prepare' themselves to stammer. He called this preparation an abnormal 'preparatory set', which, having been initiated, virtually ensures that the person will go on to stammer (Van Riper, 1973). The goal of block modification is therefore for the person to learn a new motor preparatory set to use in place of the abnormal one. Ward (2006) refers to modification as 'the phase of therapy where "abnormal" stuttering is changed into a less effortful version' (p249).

When to use

- For modification to be effective, the client must have closely identified what it is he does when he stammers (see Chapter 5 'Identification').

- He must also be sufficiently desensitised to his stammering.

- In addition, the client needs to have a sufficient number of at least moderately severe blocks for this technique to be worthwhile for him.

- We also suggest that the 'backtracker' needs to do some preliminary work before starting block modification. The backtracker is a person who approaches a difficult word and then goes back and repeats one or more words as a run-in. We feel that the person with this type of stammer should be helped to 'move forward' in his speech before learning block modification. He can do this by a combination of identification, monitoring and reminders by others.

- In our view, the client also needs to have had some experimentation with change, both in non-speech and speech (see Chapter 4 'Variation: non-speech and speech').

Manning points out that modification is not easy to achieve: 'The old patterns are not only well-learned, they are comfortable. The new, better ways of speaking will feel awkward and strange, at least until they are practised enough to become habituated' (2000, p284).

We believe that personal understanding of how an individual reacts to change, how he feels others react, and some experimentation in changing aspects of speech (such as slowing down the rate, using lighter contacts and so on) are, therefore, an essential foundation for being able to modify the stammer (see Chapter 4).

Teaching block modification

Block modification is taught in three phases which are practised 'backwards', starting after the block has occurred and moving to before the block has started. The three phases are called cancellation (post-block modification), pull-outs (in-block modification) and pre-sets (pre-block modification). It is crucial that adequate time is spent on each phase before the client moves on to the next one. Cancellation is seen as the most important of the stages as it forms the foundation on which the others are built. Consequently, more therapy time will be spent on this stage than on any other.

The processes of block modification are illustrated in Figure 14.1.

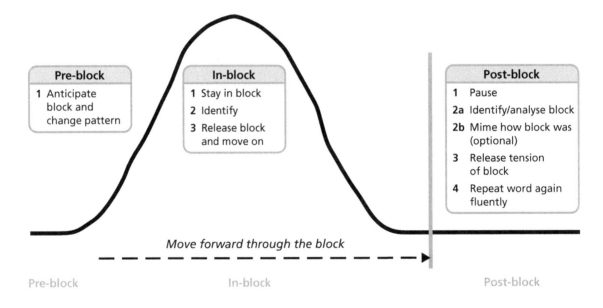

Figure 14.1 Block modification

Stage 1 Cancellation/post-block modification

Van Riper sums up the advantages of cancellation as follows:

> The stutterer needs to slay his dragon not once but many times. Every time he stutters he has a new opportunity to do so again. He has a new sense of self mastery and esteem. He has learned that he need not yield helplessly when feared words or situations come his way, that he need not struggle randomly. He has something specific to do and this in itself tends to counteract ambivalence and panic. Each cancellation is a frank admission of his stuttering; there is no denial, no disguise to leave the residue of guilt.
> (1973, p327)

In this phase the stammer is modified after it has occurred. Bloodstein (1995) describes this as cancelling failures. Van Riper developed cancellation as a sort of safety net, a way in which the stammer could still be modified even if the person had been unable to use a more normal preparatory set. Van Riper (1973) proposed that cancellation prevents the self-reinforcement of stammering. When the person stammers through a word he achieves his aim of finally finishing the word and gets nearer to the goal of 'communication closure'. Usually, he then receives a 'pay-off' in terms of several words of fluency. Cancellation does not allow him this reward and therefore this pay-off is 'cancelled out'. In addition, cancellation brings the person into close proximity to his stammer; as he confronts it his purpose is to understand *exactly* what is happening during the stammering.

Processes in cancellation

Pausing

The person is instructed to stammer through the word in his usual way and, once it is completed, to pause for about three seconds. (Van Riper, in recognising the tendency for people to underestimate how long this is, suggests they count three hippopotamuses! Others suggest the more conventional 'one thousand, two thousand, three thousand'.) The stammered word must be finished to lessen the likelihood of repeated attempts at the word or 'run-ins' and to keep the person moving forward in his speech. Pausing after stammering is rarely easy for several reasons. When a person stammers he often fears pauses in his speech and therefore we are asking him now to do something that he may not only have deliberately avoided for many years but may not have perceived as helpful in maintaining fluency. In addition, it is a difficult task for a person to recognise all his stammers in time to cancel them, even when he is being extremely vigilant. We find it is best to ask clients to start by 'getting hold of' their most severe stammers. Sometimes people find it helpful to give descriptive names to these stammers; one client called them 'sharks' – because they are big, vicious and dangerous. The client is usually more aware of these severe stammers; they are thus easier to cancel and he gets a feeling of success for doing so. Once he can cancel most of the severe stammers, he can move on to attempt to cancel less severe ones.

Using the pause for relaxation and identification

As soon as the client is able to use the pause after a reasonable number of his stammers (perhaps around 50 per cent, but this will vary between individuals), he is asked to use the pause to calm himself and to let go of any tension in his body before he continues with the next word. Van Riper (1973) points out that it is easier for a client to relax after a stammer than before or during it. In addition, the listener is more likely to react favourably when the client appears to be taking control of his stammering. Once the client can do this fairly easily, he moves on to use the pause to identify exactly what he is doing when he stammers, in preparation for the next stage of cancellation.

Reduplicating the stammer

This next process is not always easy to 'sell' to a client, even when he understands and agrees with the rationale. This is because it confronts his stammering behaviour 'head on'. The person is asked to reduplicate in pantomime the stammer he has just performed, that is, to silently perform the stammer again, exactly as it occurred originally. If, for example, he pushed his lips together and his head forward, then this is what he will repeat. The person, therefore, has to do again that very thing he fears. In doing so, he becomes aware of exactly what he did to bring the stammer into being. In the process he learns that stammering is something he *does*. Although Van Riper advocates that the reduplication should be pantomimed (that is, without

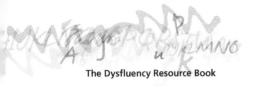

voice, as a 'mime'), we find there are some people for whom the onset of voicing is so crucial in the stammering behaviour that the reduplication needs to be *exactly* like the original (that is, with phonation). Clearly, this phase is rarely easy to do and sometimes too difficult to consider in some situations: for example, in a bus queue in the rush hour! Clients are encouraged to use reduplication in situations they find easiest. These are often situations with people to whom they can explain what is happening and with whom they can be sure they will have the time they need to carry out the process without pressure to finish the word quickly.

Reduplicating the word in a more fluent way

In this stage the person again pantomimes the stammered word but follows this by doing so in a new, slower and improved way. To use the example from the last section, this time the person repeats the word with his lips gently put together and his head remaining in the mid-line. He is not merely saying the word again and 'happening' to be fluent; he is actually doing something, in the way he shapes his mouth, relaxes his speech organs and so on, which will give him more control. What he does is based on what he has learned through identification, pausing and pantomiming. He is now correcting the motor movements or 'sets'. Once again, he needs to choose carefully the situations in which it is most feasible to carry out this process.

Saying the word again more fluently

This is the final process in cancellation. The person stammers, pauses and repeats the word in his new way, no longer pantomiming the stammered word first. The repetition is now said aloud. Thus the process goes: stammered word, pause, word resaid in a more fluent way.

Some clients do not move on from this stage of modification as they feel that cancellation alone gives them enough control. For others, cancellation is just the first step in the process. We believe it is important to tailor the therapy to the client, not the client to the therapy. Thus, while there are some guiding principles, both client and clinician need to experiment to help the client find what is most useful for *him*.

Problems that can occur during this stage

- Levy (1987) warns against the use of cancellation with interiorised stammerers. She states that cancellation runs contrary to the aim of therapy with this group, which is to stammer openly rather than to control the stammering. However, she notes that some clients find full cancellation useful and also that it may be a suitable procedure for those who cannot succeed with pre-sets or pull-outs.

- Sometimes a client may find it especially hard to get hold of his stammers because he is used to rushing on from them at great speed. We have found it useful to introduce an intermediate step for such a person. We suggest that he tries to 'walk away' rather than 'run away' from the stammer; in other words, as soon as he is aware of what is happening he aims to slow down the next few words as a first phase of taking control. It can be helpful for him to tell others what he is doing in order to ensure that he is given adequate time to carry out the cancellation procedure. This can be especially important on the telephone, where listeners have no non-verbal clues to inform them that the conversation is still in progress.

- Other possible problems of cancellation are shown in Table 14.1.

Table 14.1 Possible problems in the cancellation/post-block phase

Problem	Possible solutions
1 The client does not have any major blocks – the blocks are all mild and difficult to 'catch'	The client may not need therapy
	Block modification may not be the treatment of choice
	Further monitoring may be required
	Encourage the client to start by walking away from block (see the second bullet point above)
	Work alongside the client and model what he is aiming for
	Increase work on desensitisation
2 The client pauses during the stammer, before completing the stammered word	Explain the need to move forward in speaking, not to revise what has already been said; this will make speaking sound more normal
3 The client does not pause for long enough after the block	Check that the client understands the rationale for the length of pause
	Do further desensitisation work on tolerating pausing and silence (see Chapter 7)
	Model pausing with the client
	Help the client to practise in non-emotive conversations
	Enlist the help of a significant other who can remind the client
	Use the 'hippopotamuses' to help the client judge the length of the pause more accurately and to 'let go' of the urgency of conversation
4 The listener interrupts during the pause	The speaker explains what he is doing where possible
	The speaker uses a non-verbal signal (eg eye contact or touch) to show that he has not yet finished speaking
	The speaker continues to speak over the listener
5 The client wants to move on to in-block modification too soon	The client will probably try to do so regardless of advice from the clinician!
	Ensure that if this fails, the client uses post-block as a 'safety net'

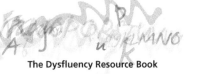
Problem	Possible solutions
6 The client needs to repeat the stammer aloud, rather than pantomime, in order to be able to identify what he is doing (eg the onset of voicing may be a crucial part of the stammer and can only be identified properly if reduplicated)	Let him! This may well be the only way he can work out what is happening
7 The client will not pantomime the stammer and/or the new way of saying the word	Try to persuade the client to do this in the clinical setting, and if possible in one very safe situation outside, to get the feel of what is going wrong and how to change it Discuss the advantages of this with a client who has found it helpful

Stage 2 Pull-outs/in-block modification

The next stage involves modifying the stammer as it is happening. The client is staying with the stammer but taking hold of it rather sooner than in cancellation, identifying what is happening as it happens, and learning to release it under his control. This stage should not be commenced until the client is able to cancel a majority of his stammers. Van Riper (1973) points out that frequently, once someone is proficient at cancellation, he often starts this next process by himself, without instruction. The eventual aim of pull-outs is fluent stammering, but any change in the abnormal pattern that is being produced should be considered a positive step. Luper and Mulder (1964) use an analogy which a client may find helpful. They compare pull-outs to releasing oneself from a bramble, saying that if it gets stuck on your clothing:

> you may get snagged tightly, skin and clothes, if you try to jerk free. There is little real danger to be found in a blackberry patch if you proceed carefully, but you may be in for some real trouble if you panic. Whether entangled in a blackberry patch or in a stuttering block, the only danger comes through losing your head.
> (1964, p135)

The clinician encourages the client to experiment with his own ways of pulling out but can also demonstrate some ways of dealing with specific sorts of stammering behaviours that others have found helpful.

Dealing with blocks

This starts by continuing and slowing down the stammering behaviour. The articulators can then be moved into a more normal position if necessary (for example, releasing the tongue from a tense closure with the palate), before moving into the position needed for the following sound. An example might be as follows: the client blocks on the 'g' of 'gather'. In doing so, he not only presses the back of his tongue tightly against his palate, but also pushes the edge of his tongue against the side of his teeth. In addition, his eyebrows are raised. 'Pulling out' involves slowing down the sound (so that it becomes more like a fricative in nature), releasing the side of the tongue from the teeth and forming the mouth into the shape needed to make the vowel sound 'a'. The eyebrows are lowered.

An alternative way of dealing with a block could be to change it gradually into a repetition. For example, the client blocks on 'p' in 'paper'; he changes it from a hard block to 'p, p, pay, pay, paper'.

Van Riper (1973) makes some special suggestions for silent blocks occurring at a laryngeal level. He recommends the use of vocal fry (creaky voice) to make the transition from silence to phonation and air flow. The first phase involves intermittent vocal fry, changing in the next phase to making it continuous. Phase three combines the use of vocal fry with real phonation before moving on to the final phase of real phonation and no fry. In time the person learns to reduce the number of steps he needs to take in this process.

The clinician's task at this stage is to ensure that the client closely examines what he is doing, so that he learns correct procedures from the outset. He needs to be constantly reminded when he fails to carry out a procedure and to be given constructive feedback on his handling of the stammer. The clinician must be both able and prepared to model techniques and to answer queries as they arise.

Dealing with prolongations

Here the essence of pulling out is moving on in the word, past the sound the client is sticking on. The client finds the appropriate movement he has to make in order to do this. In addition to releasing any associated tension, this may involve making a different articulatory contact, such as moving the tongue tip back for the movement from 's' to 'l' or a new mouth shape if moving on to a vowel sound.

Dealing with repetitions

Slowing down the rate at which repetitions are produced and releasing any associated tension helps the client to take control of the stammer before moving on to the next sound in the word. It may also be necessary to move from the inclusion of the 'schwa' vowel to the vowel which is appropriate for the word. Alternatively, the repetition can be changed into a prolongation which is under the person's control as he eases out of the stammer altogether.

Where pull-outs of the stammer are unsuccessful, or only partly successful, it is suggested that the client returns to cancelling the word. In this way he is always doing something constructive about his stammering.

Table 14.2 Possible problems in the pull-out/in-block phase

Problem	Possible solutions
1 The client wants to proceed to pre-block modification too quickly	Explain again the rationale for mastering each stage of modification before moving to the next one
	Explain that he may fail, but let him try
	Ensure that any failures are cancelled
	Agree a set of situations in which he can do this, but identify another set in which he continues to use post-block modification

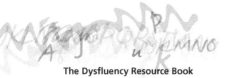

Problem	Possible solutions
2 The client misses out this phase altogether	Let him do so, but teach pull-outs as a safety net for failures
	Help the client to use this phase in the clinic or at home in reading or word lists
	Encourage him to discuss this with another client, preferably one who has overcome a similar problem
	Ask the client to write a list of advantages and disadvantages of in-block modification for now and for the future
	Parallel pull-outs with the client
3 The client only uses pull-outs with certain kinds of stammer	Suggest that the client cancels these other blocks, but encourage continued work on pull-outs

Stage 3 Pre-sets/pre-block modification

This is the final stage of block modification. Again, it is common for a client to start this stage by himself as he becomes increasingly competent at pulling out of his stammers.

Van Riper (1973) sees pre-block modification as a new way of approaching those very signals that previously had triggered struggle and avoidance behaviours. It involves planning a new way of starting and continuing the word by slowing it down and making smooth transitions between sounds. In essence, the client is replacing his old way of stammering with the new way he has found through post-block and in-block modification. Van Riper (1973) suggests that the person starts by introducing the fluent stammers into his speech on non-feared words as a way of seeing how little a listener is likely to notice and how little the process interferes with communication. He can then move on to using pre-sets on feared words.

The process involves pausing before an anticipated stammer in order to relax the speech muscles. The person then plans how to execute the speech movements in a new way before proceeding to say the word: 'I need to place my lips together loosely in order to make the "p" sound and to keep my head in the mid-line as I do so'. It is important to keep the production of the word slow and controlled. In due course the person may be able to leave out the pause as he becomes more proficient at using this technique and it becomes more automatic.

It is very important to warn the client that the pause is to be used for relaxation and planning and not for postponement, as this may be a temptation. He also needs to be sure to use in-block modification if pre-sets fail and to use cancellation if he does not cope successfully with in-blocks. In this way he is still always working on the stammered word in a positive way.

Table 14.3 Possible problems in the pre-set/pre-block phase

Problem	Possible solutions
1 The client moves himself to this stage without having learned in-block modification	Suggest that he goes back to learn in-block as this will be something he can fall back on if his attempts at pre-block fail
2 The client cannot 'catch' the stammer before it occurs	Spend time helping the client to 'catch' the stammer first without trying to modify it, by just pausing as soon as he becomes or is made aware of it
3 The client uses the pause as a postponement device	Explain why this is counter-productive Do more desensitisation work

Other problems that can occur in learning block modification

1 The client has previously learned another technique and it is incompatible with block modification. An example of this might be a client who has learned easy onset and can use it well at the beginning of an utterance. Clinician and client need to work together to decide how to integrate the two techniques. One solution in this case could be for the client to use block modification on the more severe stammers and easy onset on the less severe ones.

2 The client will only use block modification in a limited range of situations, for example, in speech and language therapy sessions or at home. Clinicians can help to extend the range of situations by:

- bringing along a former client who has experienced similar anxieties to discuss how he managed to get over them

- inviting the client to bring someone from their home environment into the clinic to demonstrate the process to them and enlist their help in transfer

- the clinician herself 'faking' block modification in a public setting to allow the client to observe the reaction of others

- giving the client time to feel confident about his ability to use the technique and then using a hierarchy to very gradually extend the situations in which it is used.

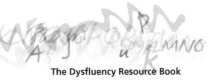
Activities for block modification

Clients need to feel confident in their ability to use block modification in the clinic, at home, when reading or with someone they are close to before taking it into the outside environment. In the clinical setting they are encouraged to use block modification as often as possible. Its use is closely monitored by the clinician and appropriate feedback is given.

Using printed material as basis for discussion ⓘ ⚙

The client reads and discusses with the clinician and/or group members Handout 45 'Block modification' and, if appropriate, other written information about the technique. We have found Fraser (2007) to be particularly useful as it guides clients through the process step by step.

Modelling ⓘ ⚙

The clinician and/or an ex-client demonstrate the different phases of block modification. Ex-clients may be able to demonstrate actual stammering, whereas the clinician will have to 'fake' stammering in a similar way to the client. This process is likely to be helpful at each of the three phases of block modification.

Use of visual recording ⓘ

It can be helpful for clients to see their attempts – good and bad – at using block modification and to analyse what went well and what else they could have done when they stammered.

Problem discussion ⓘ ⚙

An ex-client is asked to talk to the client(s) and discuss problems the client(s) may be having. It may feel easier for the client to take advice from someone who has been through many of the same struggles as him than from a clinician who can never know exactly what it is like to learn and use the technique.

Conversation with the clinician and/or group members ⓘ ⚙

The client is required to cancel as many stammers as he can, while the clinician (or group members) counts both the modified and unmodified blocks. The client aims to make the ratio of modified blocks greater than unmodified ones in successive practices. Once the client is modifying most blocks in simple conversation, increasingly difficult conversational situations can be used. Some ideas for introducing complexity might be:

- emotional topics: for example, things that make people happy, sad and so on, the best or worst day of my life

- complex descriptions: for example, how to change a tyre, sew on a button, make a lasagne

- difficult listener reactions: for example, being interrupted, asked a lot of questions, being talked to very quickly.

Instructing the clinician ⓘ

Van Riper (1973) suggests a useful activity for the pull-out phase. The clinician fakes a stammer similar to that of the client and the client then tells her what to do in order to pull out from it. This may involve demonstrations by the client in order that the clinician is sure of what to do.

Helping the analysis ⓘ

The clinician can help the client in the analysis of his blocks, especially in the in-block phase, by signalling to him to hold on to his articulatory and respiratory posture. For example, a finger or clenched fist may indicate to the client to 'freeze', and then, after a few seconds, release of the postures can be signalled by lowering the finger or gently unclenching the fist. During the 'freezing' the clinician can talk the client through his analysis and direct his attention to various aspects of his block.

Although somewhat out of sync, this technique may also be used *before* cancellation begins as a way of introducing a client to what he needs to be doing during his pause once the block has ended.

Outside assignments ⓘ

The clinician can accompany the client on outside assignments, watch him use techniques and give appropriate feedback.

Home-based activity

The client is asked to 'collect' numbers of modified and unmodified stammers in a specified time span and with a variety of listeners. Some clients find it helpful to use a hierarchy to gradually increase the complexity of the task. Others prefer to use the techniques in as many situations as possible from the start.

Block modification

So far in your therapy you have:

- identified the various component parts of your overt and covert stammer (what others see and hear and what is hidden from them)
- begun to change the way you feel about yourself and your stammer (desensitisation)
- experimented with changing things about yourself and your communication (variation)
- reduced some of your avoidances.

Now you are ready to start to change the stammer itself. The aim of this part of therapy is not for you to become completely fluent, but for you to be able to change the way you stammer and to feel that you have control. This has been called 'fluent stammering'.

Block modification is divided into three stages: (1) cancellation or post-block modification, (2) pull-outs or in-block modification, and (3) pre-sets or pre-block modification. We start work on modifying or changing the stammer *after* it has occurred and work backwards, modifying it *during* the word next and finally *before* the word. This may sound rather strange but we do it because it is easier to approach it in this way.

Cancellation/post-block modification

In this phase you learn first to 'catch' and then to 'take hold of' the stammer once it has occurred. This is no easy task and takes a lot of determination and practice. Having struggled through a block, you will probably find that, like most people, you just want to carry on speaking. In addition, after blocking, you may find you are 'rewarded' by several words of fluency. This tends to make it more likely that you will again push through the next difficult word; in other words it reinforces the stammering. This is because you know that after pushing through the word you will not only get some relief, but also some fluency. Cancellation breaks that link by preventing you from getting the fluency reward. It makes you stay with the stammer, not run away from it as you have done in the past. As the name implies, it cancels out the stammer because you are now doing something positive about it. There are several stages in cancellation:

1 Finish the stammered word in any way you can. Do not go back and start it again. Immediately after finishing it, pause for three seconds. This is longer than you might think. Do not rush the pause. If you find it difficult to pause (and most people find it takes a while to be able to do it consistently), you may find it helpful to add another stage instead. This involves 'walking away' from the block. If you cannot pause, then try to say the next few words particularly slowly, rather than rushing them out. Once you have learned to catch blocks in this way, you will start to find it easier to pause immediately after the block, as described above.

2 Use the pause to really calm down and relax, getting rid of all the tension associated with the stammer. Become aware of this tension and how it feels to let it go. You might, for example, notice if your lips are pushed together or if your tongue is moving quickly against the roof of your mouth. You might become aware that your head moves forward or your eyes close.

Continued on Handout 45.2 →

3   In the pause reproduce your stammer as it was, but silently. This is called 'pantomiming'. Try to repeat exactly what happened in the block; in this way you are learning more about your stammer – what you actually do and how it feels – in preparation for changing it.

4   This time, in addition to 'pantomiming' the stammer as it was, you 'pantomime' a new, more fluent way of saying it, without all the struggle that went on in your first attempt.

5   The final stage of cancellation involves just repeating the stammered word aloud after the pause, this time in a slow, controlled way.

Pull-outs/in-block modification

In this next phase you take control of the stammer as it occurs and change the way it proceeds. You need to take action as soon as you can after the stammer has started. Do not continue to push through the word, but instead hold on to the stammer as you think through the movements you need to make to complete the word in a new, more fluent way. You will have learned a lot about what you need to do through identification and the pantomiming work you did in cancellation. Different sorts of stammer will benefit from different sorts of pull-out. We give a few examples here but suggest you look at strategies for pulling out of your own stammer with your clinician.

Dealing with blocks where you make some sound

Slow the block down and release all the tension connected with it. For example, if you block on a 'b' sound, extend the sound as you release all the tension around your lips. Look towards the next sound in the word as you do this and make the mouth shape required for it. If, for example, the word is 'bean', you will need to open your mouth and widen it (rather as you do when you smile). Another way of pulling out of blocks is to gradually turn them into repetitions and reduce the tension with each repetition. Thus the word 'bean' might sound as follows: 'b, b, b, bean'.

Dealing with blocks where there is no sound

For these stammers, which occur at your larynx (voice box), the task involves first producing some sound. As you let go of the tension, the aim is to produce what is known as 'creaky voice'. This releases air through the vocal cords. Once this has happened, you can start to produce some normal sound. You will need to experiment with your clinician over the stages you may need to go through before you will be able to complete the word. (We would not suggest you try to use 'creaky voice' without talking to the clinician first; it is all too easy to get into bad habits which then have to be unlearned!)

Dealing with repetitions

These stammers essentially need to be slowed down and made in an increasingly relaxed way. How many repetitions you need to do at the increasingly slower speed will depend on the amount of tension that is present and the rate at which you are able to let it go. As you get more experienced at doing this, the process will probably take less time. The aim is to keep slowing the repetitions down until you feel in control.

Continued on Handout **45.3** →

H45.2

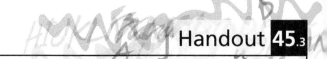

Pre-sets/pre-block modification

This is the final stage of block modification. Here you anticipate a stammer and deal with it in advance in order to reduce its intensity. You need to be aware that you are going to stammer in order to do this. The stages are as follows:

• Pause before the word on which you anticipate stammering.

• Relax your speech muscles, as you have learned in cancellation.

• Think of how to produce the first sound in a more fluent way (remember what you have learned in the previous phases of modification).

• Start to say the word in this new way and go on to complete the rest of the word in a slow, controlled fashion.

In due course you may be able to leave out the pause. Do not try to do this too early. When you feel ready to do so, do it gradually.

NB It is important to use the pause for relaxation and planning, not as a way of postponing or avoiding the stammer.

Remember: you have built in safety nets so that whatever happens you have done something constructive about your stammer. If you are unable to use pre-sets, use pull-outs. If you do not succeed with these, you can cancel.

Routledge This page may be photocopied for instructional use only. *The Dysfluency Resource Book* © J Turnbull & T Stewart 2010

15 | Maintenance: a continuing process of change

Since writing the first edition of *The Dysfluency Resource Book,* we have elaborated our approach to 'maintenance' significantly. Rather than seeing maintenance as a stage that happens at the end of therapy, we see it as a process that actually begins from the first session with a client. From day one we encourage clients to identify, develop and consistently use a range of 'tools' or strategies. This collection of tools, having been gathered and honed during therapy, will then equip a client for the often demanding situations and events that happen in the future. The toolbox must have certain design features:

1   The toolbox will have more than a 'maintenance' function: it will equip the individual with the capacity to cope with change.

2   The toolbox will be filled with dynamic strategies, 'tools' that are flexible and meet the needs of the person at a given moment, whatever they may be. A box of techniques, for example, containing only suggestions for controlling fluency, would not be adaptable enough to cope with this demand for flexibility. (We learned this from our clients when we asked them what strategies they were using some months or years after the end of therapy (Stewart & Richardson, 2004).)

3   The tools will not just relate to fluency or communication (although some may) but will be wide-ranging and holistic, providing the client with the means to manage his thoughts, feelings and behaviours.

When to use

As stated previously, we see the process of maintenance as starting at the beginning of therapy. We encourage each client to purchase a special notebook to bring to therapy in which he will record the tools as he identifies and collects them. This forms his own record of time in therapy and will enable him to write a summary of his toolbox before he leaves the clinic setting. In group or individual intervention the person reads his toolbox aloud as a way of marking the outcomes of therapy and creating a point of closure from this stage of change. In addition, we ask the client to invite a significant person in his life to come and 'witness' his toolbox. This person will then be a link with the use of these strategies in the situations that lie ahead.

Readers may wonder what strategies a client could gather from the various principles of therapy we have outlined in previous chapters. Here are some examples.

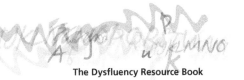

Identification

- Skills to help ongoing monitoring of speech (for example, rate, tension) and non-speech aspects of his life (for example, levels of stress).
- The ability to recognise the need to instigate a change (for example, to slow the pace of life).

Desensitisation

- The need to be open with new people about his stammer.
- Recognising the ongoing need to keep mentioning his stammer in situations where occasionally he has some anxieties about it.

Avoidance reduction

- Seeking out situations he does not encounter regularly so that potential fear is kept under control (for example, asking for items in shops).
- Working on areas of his life in which he feels uncomfortable about his speech (for example, expressing emotions).

Fluency control

- Working on naturalness of easy onset in conversations and requests for feedback.
- Practising techniques in a structured way from time to time to make sure they continue to be effective when and if they are required (for example, when reading, in spontaneous speech from sentence level to conversations).

Common problems

There are a number of issues that can create difficulties for clients trying to do things differently. We list them below and are aware that many of them need to be addressed before the client leaves therapy.

A client is trying out and taking on new roles. He will be involved in more speaking situations, asserting his right to speak in situations where he has been silent in the past.

Significant others. Important people in the client's life may be disconcerted by the changes he is making. This may require some adjustment on their part, for example, having to learn not to do things for the person who stammers, giving him the space to try things out or taking a back seat in situations where they would previously have taken a lead.

Monitoring. A client will need to have skills with which to monitor and identify problems as well as put remedial strategies into place. He will need to be self-reliant rather than rely on his therapist or other therapy group members.

Pressure. With increased control over speech come increased demands and expectations from others and from the client himself.

Return of old habits. 'Old habits die hard' is a saying with relevance here. There will be strong associations and triggers that will exert pressure on the client to return to old ways. The client needs to have a number of 'resistance' strategies.

Fluency necessitates faster processing time. When a client is stammering, this creates time for him to process his language production. Once those dysfluent episodes are minimised, that processing time is reduced. A client may need to have different ways of coping with this side effect of increased fluency.

Support. Leaving therapy, especially group therapy, can mean that a client loses a social network and this may create a bit of a vacuum. An alternative or different social network will need to be in place to support his ongoing progress.

Therapy as motivator. Attending regular therapy can act as a motivator for an individual. Once the need for appointments has disappeared, he will need other sources of motivation.

Relaxation. Often clients who leave therapy experience a period of 'letting go'. They enjoy not having to complete tasks or targets and can settle back into not thinking about their speech. This phase is a natural reaction following months of work. Clients need to be prepared for this and have strategies in place to help them re-engage with a process of monitoring and positive management strategies.

The client is not empowered to work autonomously on his communication. Fundamental to maintenance and continuing progress is the ability of the client to be his own expert in managing his speech. As we discussed in Chapter 1 'Principles of therapy', we develop this notion throughout the course of therapy so that clients leave with a well-developed understanding of their competencies and confidence in their own abilities.

Developing a toolbox

When a client reaches the point in therapy where he feels ready to write a summary of his toolbox, he often feels overwhelmed by the task. He may have collected several pages of notes and be unsure how to collate them into a usable format. At this stage we support his thinking by giving him some ideas about headings he might use. Examples of headings are presented below and on Handout 46 'Grid for a toolbox'.

• Tools for everyday use

• Tools for weekly use

• Tools for occasional use

• Tools to be reviewed periodically (for example, monthly, annually)

• Tools I need to practise

• Tools to live by

• Things to do when life is going well

• Things to remember when life is going less well

• Specific things I need to work on for specific situations

We ask clients to think about their tools in terms of things they can do, things they can think about and feelings that are useful. In this way the toolbox has a holistic quality.

Recently a client developed a novel format which we have included as an example (see Handout 47 'Emma's toolbox'). We believe this format is very accessible and enables the individual to see at a glance exactly what he should be referring to in his toolbox, and where and when. This is how Emma described the usefulness of this format:

> Having my toolbox in grid format allows me to see my tools (in bold) and current targets I am working towards in a clear and realistic format for everyday use.
> Each column explains how to use these tools and targets on different days. My toolbox can easily be updated and modified as I progress with targets and as I change. It is not static, but a dynamic and evolving entity. The title of my toolbox is important because it reflects the significant changes I have achieved through therapy.

Dynamic tools

We also hope that a client will develop a number of skills that he will be able to use in the future. Rather than behaviours that he learns, these are strategies which enable him to move and adapt to circumstances as they arise. Here are one or two strategies that clients have identified as useful to their 'maintenance' stage.

Problem solving

In order for a client to successfully maintain his therapy gains, he must reach a stage where he can almost be his own clinician. One factor in this process is the ability to recognise a difficulty when it arises and to critically analyse the options open to him to solve it. Thus, he should be able to examine the factors that have precipitated the obstacle, come up with a range of alternative solutions, experiment with the options he needs to check out practically, evaluate the results of his experimentation objectively and, finally, implement his preferred solution over time. This problem-solving approach should be developed and nurtured during a client's therapy programme. There are a number of key stages to problem solving (see Handout 48).

Identify or define the problem. This needs to be done in detailed behavioural terms. For example, it is not enough to say, 'I cannot use the phone'. The problem must be stated in precise detail: where the problem occurs, what time of day, who it involves, and so on. So, continuing with the example, a client may state the problem as, 'I cannot pick the receiver up, dial the doctor's/dentist's number, say hello and my name and ask for an appointment without high levels of anxiety and fear of stammering'.

Develop options for tackling the problem. One approach would be to do a brainstorming exercise. This should be carried out with an open mind. At this stage no evaluation of the advantages or disadvantages of each option is made by the client or the clinician. It is simply a gathering or collection of the possibilities.

Option appraisal. At this point the various merits and demerits of each idea are considered. This will include the predicted outcomes as well as how the client feels about the individual options. Sometimes the emotional response outweighs the more objective 'pros and cons' evaluations and therefore it is essential that this be given a high profile.

Ranking. The client puts the options in his order of preference.

Experimentation. Some of the options may need testing to see whether the outcome is as the client predicts. At this stage the client can choose to carry out this experimentation before formulating an action plan. Each experiment will be evaluated and key learning points identified.

Formulate an action plan. Having tested the options, the client is now ready to devise his plan for solving the problem. It should be made clear to him that, even at this stage, the plan should itself be regarded as an experiment, and can be modified on the basis of experience.

Put the action plan in place. The client should decide on a start date and stick to it. He may wish to consider telling another person about his plan at this point. This should ensure he does not prevaricate and that he moves ahead into the action phase.

Re-evaluate and re-plan. In order that the client takes account of his experience with the strategy, it is important that a review time is included in his plan. At this point he should reassess the effectiveness of his preferred option, consider what he has learned as a result of this approach and decide whether or not any changes are required. He may then go back to experimentation, or he could reformulate his action plan or continue with the original one as appropriate.

Use of hierarchies

Very often a client will find the task of changing something about himself daunting. However, when the task is broken down into a series of small, manageable steps it appears more achievable. Each step can be tackled in its own right, with the client focusing on the 'bite sized chunk' rather than the whole banquet! In this way, progress is made and change becomes more attainable rather than something that is always out of reach.

In therapy clients learn how to break change into smaller steps through the use of hierarchies and this skill can help them to manage difficulties more easily in the future. Handout 49 'A sample hierarchy' is a helpful guide to facilitate this learning.

Developing positive thinking

Sometimes a client's thinking can impede his ability to move forward. For example, he may predict certain outcomes and this will limit his capacity to do things differently: for example, 'I have always stammered in this situation, nothing has changed, I am going to stammer again', or 'Today is a bad day, I just know my speech will be awful'. Alternatively, a client may generalise too readily; he perhaps stammers on one word of greeting and on that basis determines that his speech is going to be dysfluent for the remainder of the conversation or even the rest of the day! Other examples of disruptive thoughts are those relating to self-esteem ('I'm hopeless at this') and other people ('He must think I am stupid'). They can be based on the short term ('This word always gives me trouble') or on longer-term outcomes ('I am going to hate myself once this is over').

We have a number of strategies that we suggest to clients to try to counteract the effects of these negative cognitions. These include:

• having a trigger thought that encourages more positive thinking ('I can always TRY and see what happens')

• focusing on the present moment: the thoughts, feelings and sensations experienced in the moment

• trying to have a balance of thoughts, both negative and positive

• confronting fears rather than avoiding them

• using rewards

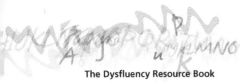

- using positive self-talk
- thinking of self as a whole person rather than 'a stammerer'
- construing self as someone who can control his speech.

Clinicians can explore other examples with clients using Handout 50 'Strategies for developing positive thinking'.

Using triggers

Triggers are little reminders, deliberately positioned to help the client remember particular strategies in situations in which he finds it difficult to recall them. A trigger can be anything that reminds the client. In the past our clients have been very inventive; they have used stickers on the phone, put a particular message on their computer screensaver, worn an elastic band on their wrist in a meeting, put their watch on the non-preferred wrist, set the alarm on their digital watch or mobile phone every hour or so; the list is as long as the number of clients. It is, of course, preferable if a client chooses his own reminders; this is more likely to ensure their effectiveness. In group therapy, other clients can often offer a range of ideas that they have found useful. A client can find it helpful to use these 'tried and tested' ideas developed by individuals who have needed to use triggers in certain situations.

Taking care of the whole person

We know that a number of factors cause clients to experience a loss of control over their speech. Illness, fatigue and stress all influence everyone to a certain degree and can also lead to changes in dysfluency. It will not be enough for an individual to develop a number of fluency-enhancing behaviours or skills if other fluency disruptors are ignored. The client needs to see his speech difficulties in the context of his whole self, and include lifestyle issues. If these are important to the individual he can be helped to develop changes in his life style, or at least experiment with different aspects of his life to see if these changes have a positive effect on his speech; they could also have a bearing on maintenance.
Factors to consider include:

- exercise
- sleep patterns
- diet
- relaxation
- alcohol and substance abuse
- general stress management.

Support networks

Although at first sight this doesn't appear like a 'tool', our clinical experience and research (Stewart & Richardson, 2004) has shown the issue of support to be an important factor in the maintenance of progress in therapy. Support comes from various sources.

Significant other involvement

Clients need the help and support of at least one other person in their lives to help them in the process of change and beyond. It is important at the outset of therapy for clinicians to inform and involve significant others for this reason (with the client's permission, of course). We ask each client to bring another person along to at least one therapy session. During this session we explain the process and the management of speech change, and the likely implications for them as someone who is close to the client, in whatever context. These visitors are welcomed at other sessions and, as we have stated previously, they are an integral part of the closure or leaving of therapy, which is marked by witnessing the client's toolbox.

Support groups
Craig (1986) assessed the effects on maintenance of regular attendance at a self-help group, regular formal practice (rate control practice alone or with a friend), performing real-life assignments regularly (tape recording performance on the telephone or a conversation) and attendance at follow-up sessions. Only attendance at the self-help group correlated mildly with long-term outcomes. While Craig is careful to emphasis the difficulty of isolating individual factors, we cannot ignore the importance of continuing support for clients at this stage.

Our experience of the local self-help group in Leeds has been a valuable adjunct to our work. With regard to maintenance issues, it proves a safe haven for a client to continue to develop and hone his toolbox. It is also a source of continuing support at a time when discharge from therapy may have meant a loss of contact with individuals who know about stammering and have a real understanding of the difficulties it can cause.

Support organisation
We recommend that each person or family who comes to see us becomes a member of the British Stammering Association. This charity is a national organisation in the UK. The Association has a book and video library, holds details of specialist clinicians and therapy courses around the country and arranges regular open days and conferences across Britain. It also produces a magazine and excellent information leaflets for parents, teachers, employers and people who stammer.

Speech/language therapy contact
We keep in contact with a client for some time after the therapy programme has ended. This open door policy enables the client to review the status of his toolbox when he needs to. This review can take place in our clinic, over the phone or, more usually these days, by email. We believe that this is an important facility to offer in view of the nature of the difficulties with maintenance, which have been well documented. In addition to structured and informal review appointments, we have offered clients individual booster sessions as necessary. We also frequently run short intensive group courses on more general communication skills (for example, assertiveness skills, construing self and fluency), which a client can choose to attend at any time.

On occasions we have had clients who have requested a specific type of long-distance contact with us. For example, one man who lived some miles from Leeds wished us to monitor his speech on an infrequent basis to 'keep it up to par'. He arranged to send us letters and/or audio tapes which we listened to, sending him feedback when we returned the tape to him. This arrangement continued until he decided he no longer needed the reassurance.

Change as an ongoing process

As we have discussed previously, our approach to maintenance is not the end of therapy but rather the beginning of another stage that will require a different type of commitment from the client. This attitude is one that we promote during therapy and we actively support the person in their ongoing monitoring, experimentation and risk taking.

Things to do	Things to think	Things to feel
Tools for everyday use		
Tools for weekly use		
Tools for occasional use		
Tools to be reviewed periodically (eg monthly, annually)		
Tools I need to practise		
Tools to live by		
Things to do when life is going well		
Things to remember when life is going less well		
Specific things I need to work on for specific situations		

Emma's toolbox

My TOOLBOX

I am supposed to stammer & I have the tools to deal with it

	Good Day Experiment, push self, step it up	Every Day Consolidate, hone and refine skills	Bad Day I have all the tools & skills I need to cope
Eye Contact	· Keep eye contact **when I stammer** to unfamiliar people	· **Initiate** & **during** interactions = good EC · Keep eye contact when I stammer	· Remember to **give it to them** bam smack between the eyes! · **Keep EC when stammer**
Relaxation – Rate	· **Call answering machine** with a long explanation to monitor rate & conciseness · **Pause**	· **3 minute** breathing space · In **moment of stammer** reduce local (relax tongue) and overall tension (feel slow all over) · **Collect** thoughts · **Pause**	· **3 minute** breathing space · Give self **time to arrive** physically & mentally · In moment of stammer reduce local (relax tongue) and overall tension (feel slow all over)
Self-advertising	· All the time – **out & proud!** · Self-advertising – practise by **creating situations** for self-advertising, i.e. introductions	· Introductions: – introduce **stammer 1st** then **name 2nd** · Generally – **commenting** on it, i.e. I have a stammer · Put it out there - **talk about stammering**	· Acknowledge that I am having a crap day and I am **only human** – everyone has them! · **Support** network – talk about it
Avoidance	<u>Word level:</u> · Tally number of fillers · Tally number of word avoidances <u>Situation level:</u> · **Choose** speaking situations · **Create** speaking opportunities – Practise phone calls	<u>Word level:</u> · Avoid use of fillers · No avoidance (re-work it in) <u>Situation level:</u> · Do **not put things off** · **Choose speaking** situations, i.e. ask for ticket, not use machine	<u>Word level:</u> · No avoidance (re-work it in) <u>Situation level:</u> · **Choose speaking** · **Grab the bull by the horns** · Do not put ANYTHING off! Phone calls, speaking to someone (look at specific situation tools)
Positive Cognitions	· Tackle unsupportive thoughts: Identification & PS approach · **Write fluency diary** (Positives)	· Read double sided **card** · Replace unhelpful thoughts with more support ones, i.e. look at **jewel card**. · **Write fluency diary** (Positives)	· Read double sided **card** · **Jewel cards** **Then -** · Write down all the good things I can think of · Read self characterization Think is there anything else that is contributing to the way I feel? Be objective, cut self some slack! · **Write fluency diary** (Positives)
Mindfulness	Thought catcher: · **Awareness** of thoughts · +/- Replace with more supportive thoughts	Thought catcher: · **Awareness** of thoughts · +/- Replace with more supportive thoughts	Thought catcher: · **Awareness** of thoughts · +/- Replace with more supportive thoughts

Continued on Handout **47.2** →

	Good Day *Experiment, push self, step it up*	**Every Day** *Consolidate, hone and refine skills*	**Bad Day** *I have all the tools & skills I need to cope*
Monitoring & Awareness	· Monitor & Review use of tools · Monitor & Review targets setting · **Write fluency diary** (Monitor)	· Identify any constructive negatives (not just being hard on myself!), analyze and take a problem solving/solution focused approach · **Write fluency diary** (Monitor)	· **Write fluency diary** (Monitor)
Post-block modification	· Use in conversation with strangers · Aim for use 100% of the time	· Use as much as I can when in general conversation, i.e. with housemates, friends etc	
Self-advertising: Introductions	· Use 100% of the time in all naturally occurring instances · Create opportunities to introduce myself, i.e. phone calls, requesting	· Introduce myself at least once (if not occur naturally make a random phone call)	
Self-advertising: Phone calls	· 3 x phone calls using self-advertising at the beginning	· 2 x phone calls using self-advertising at the beginning	

Practice Plan:

Points about practice:
· Continue LOOSENING/CHANGE
· Take risks – an active process
· Be vigilant for chances to change
· Continue to monitor

Tools:
Daily: Keep them oiled – focus on 1 tool each day to 'oil' & use all every day

Weekly: Add to my tools the steps achieved from my current targets hierarchies, i.e. using in block modification with close friends

Current targets:
Goal setting time & reviewing

1. Make a hierarchy to achieve target. Once achieved I can put it into my toolbox

2. At the **start** of each week **set a goal** based upon a level in the hierarchy & plan how to incorporate it into the coming week

3. At the **end** of each **week review** this goal. If achieved move up a level or if not break it down further

Daily Practice:

AM:

30 secs - when having breakfast
· Read double sided **card**

2 mins when packing bag
· Carry toolbox summary
· Stick **post-it** with **tool & current target**
I want to focus/work on for the day on
the front of my **diary**. Put it on my phone
background

· *GOOD day* Move up a level on the
hierarchy for that current target, i.e.
in-block modification, move from using
it with Debs to using it with close friends

Lunch:

2 mins = Read **toolbox summary**

Bed:

5 mins
· Write **fluency diary:**
  o Monitor: Current target – Context –
    Achieved?
    Or what do I need to do differently?
  o Positive: 1 x Speech specific
  o Positive: 1 x General day
· Shade in **monitoring sheet** for tool and
  target worked on that day
· Choose **tool and target** to work on
  for **tomorrow**

Specific situation:

Phone Calls: Tools = more support thoughts/desensitisation –
self-advertising & avoidance reduction: words, making call in first place

Before:
· Don't put it off. If need to do it, do it there and then
· Awareness of thoughts – 'catch' it & think what thoughts might support me better – i.e. I am
  supposed to stammer & I have the tools to deal with it

On phone:
· Self-advertising at start
· No word avoidance
· Rate control
· Use block mod

Thoughts that might support me better:
o *I am supposed to stammer & I have the tools to deal with it *
o I have had some calls that have been fine – I may have stammered but I did get my message
  across & person on other end was fine, understanding, OK
o It's OK to stammer – it doesn't always need to get in the way of the call
o I can take the time I need
o It is possible for stammering to co-exist with giving a good impression

Problem solving

1 Define the problem ....

2 What causes the problem to happen? ....

3 Was there a time when the problem was absent? Was there a time when I was able to lessen/reduce/solve the problem?
....

   What did I do? ....

   What happened? ....

   Was anyone else involved? ....

   What did I learn from this? ....

   Can I apply anything from that situation to help me with the current difficulty?

   ....

4 Make a list of all the possible ways of solving this problem

   Option A ....

   Option B ....

   Option C ....

5 Write a plan for how I am going to test out the usefulness of the options listed above

   Step 1 ....

   Step 2 ....

   Step 3 ....

   Step 4 ....

   Step 5 ....

   Add more if necessary

Routledge

Continued on Handout **48.**2 ➜

6   Results of trying out options

Results from option A ....

Results from option B ....

Results from option C ....

7   What have I learned from testing out these options?...

....

....

8   Write my action plan for solving this problem

I am going to: ....

....

....

9   Review the plan after a suitable time interval

What has worked? ....

What has worked less well? ....

Do I need to change my plan? ....

10 Make a note of things I have learned from this problem-solving task
I must remember:

(a) ....

(b) ....

(c) ....

(d) ....

(e) ....

Routledge
Taylor & Francis Group

A sample hierarchy

Phoning the doctor or dentist to make an appointment:

Dial the doctor/dentist. Listen to them answer the phone, say hello and your name and when you would like an appointment

Dial a friend and rehearse phoning the doctor/dentist (you will have had to explain to your friend beforehand what you intend to do)

Dial someone who you know well but who does not know about this difficulty, listen to them answer the phone, say hello and your name and have a short conversation with them

Dial someone who you have spoken to previously about this problem, listen to them answer the phone, say hello and your name and have a short conversation

Dial a friend who has an answering machine, listen to the message, say hello and your name and then replace the receiver

Dial the 'speaking clock', listen to the message, say hello and your name and then replace the receiver

Pick up the receiver every time you pass it and say hello and your name before replacing it

Pick up the phone every time you pass it and then replace the receiver

START

Strategies for developing positive thinking

1 A 'jewel card'

On a piece of card or a postcard write down a number of events, experiences, situations and/ or achievements which you recall with positive emotions. They can be anything at all: small events such as when someone once said something to you that meant a great deal, or bigger occasions such as receiving an award or prize for an achievement. These are your 'jewels'. In situations when you are aware of thinking negatively or when you are going through a bad patch generally, take out your 'jewels', your special moments, and spend some time remembering a particular event and how you felt then.

2 A 'toolbox' reminder

When things are not going so well with your speech, have a small card in your pocket with a summary of your 'tools' or strategies, skills and positive ideas written on it: for example, 'Slowing down helps me', 'Open up to stammering', 'I can communicate well even if I stammer'.

3 Concentrate on the present

Do not worry about things that may happen in the future. You can do very little about them. Focus your energies on factors that you can work on in the here and now.

4 Balance the negative thoughts with positive ones

If a negative thought comes into your head, take it out, shut it out. Then replace it with a positive one. Do not leave a space. The negative one is sure to return! For example, a negative thought might be, 'I will stammer here'; a positive thought would be, 'My communication skills are good and my message will still come over well'. Try to develop a little store of good and encouraging positive thoughts so that you can pull them out when you need them. Remember the ones that really work and make you feel good.

5 Confront the fear

When something is really bothering you and you cannot get it out of your head, then confront the fear. Ask yourself what it is exactly that is worrying you about the situation or event. Try to imagine the worst thing that could happen to you and think of all the possible actions you might take if the worst did occur. Often you will find that not only is the worst thing not so terrible, but you have strategies to deal with it.

6 Use a reward

If you have done something positive, taken a risk, tried something different, worked hard on your speech and so on, give yourself a reward. This might be some form of treat: a long hot bath, a chocolate bar or special meal, or an outing to a favourite place. If you prefer something more immediate, you could take some time out to recall something that makes you feel good. Try to remember it with lots of detail and enjoy the recollection. Telling someone else can also make it special.

Routledge
Taylor & Francis Group

Continued on Handout **50.2** →

7 Thinking about yourself positively

Think of yourself as someone with a stammer, not as a stammerer. You are not the sum total of your speech. There is much more to you than just the way you talk.

Remember you have a number of strategies which you can use to control your speech. Your speech does not have to control you.

8 Give yourself permission to stammer

If you are having a bad day with your speech, then use it as a learning experience. Don't go back to the old habits of pushing the sounds out, avoiding and so on. Look at what is happening in your life generally; it may be that your speech is a reflection of pressure, tiredness or change. Perhaps you need to make allowances for yourself and think, 'OK, it's not so good today, but that is hardly surprising given all that I have to cope with at the moment. I need to take extra care of myself and my speech and look at my toolbox to see what I should do'. Telling others too can help: for example, 'I'm having a really bad day with my speech today'.

9 Give yourself permission to worry

If you get anxious about your speech, try to leave the worrying to a specific time, for example, 7pm or on the train home from work. Then allow yourself to *worry like crazy* for a full 10–15 minutes. After this time you must stop and move on to thinking about other things.

10 Use your knowledge about stammering

Remember what you know about stammering. It is very variable; it comes and goes. Try and put the good days and the not so good days into perspective.

The Dysfluency Resource Book © J Turnbull & T Stewart 2010

16 | Working in groups

There is much research across social sciences into the importance of working in groups. It is not the remit of this book to discuss this in any depth. However, a brief summary follows.

Reducing isolation. The greatest effect of people meeting together is in reducing their feelings of isolation, irrespective of the content of the group meetings.

Support. This has an important function in the change process that occurs in therapy. Although an integral feature of group therapy, the nature of the support often happens without planning. In any group meeting clinicians should not underestimate the significance of clients meeting together, talking about issues, hearing each other and empathising.

Motivation. Regular therapy alone can be motivating. If a person attends for a session once a week, meets with a clinician and talks about what he has been trying to achieve, that in itself will spur him on. This effect can be multiplied if he has to account for himself in a group context *and* if the group consists of peers who are going through the same process.

Normalising effects. When people come together in a group they often realise that many of their experiences are not fundamentally different from those of others. This 'normalising' helps individual clients to change their perspective: for example, 'This is not quite the problem I thought it was. It is experienced by others and I can see others managing it in different ways. This gives me hope that I can do the same.'

Reducing dependence on the clinician. If managed correctly, the group can take on the expert role. In group therapy a client is able to access a wide range of knowledge and opinion, not just from the group members, but from people brought into the group, such as significant other people and individuals invited to the group. In this way the client can extend his network of support from the clinician to the group as a whole and beyond.

Introducing reality. Individual therapy tends to be safe and non-threatening. However, in a group the interaction tends to replicate real-life situations. For example, individuals interrupt each other, people disagree and sometimes experience anxiety. Also, within a group each individual will have to deal with a variety of interactions (for example, in the group, in pairs, in formal and informal presentations).

In addition to these well-documented benefits, we have found that working in groups is an efficient and effective way of managing a caseload. It also enables the clinicians to learn from each other's style of interaction, knowledge and skills. It can help in the development of less experienced clinicians and in addition, it's fun!

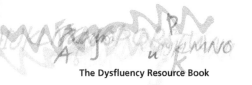

When to use

'Groups available for all.' We are firm believers in group therapy as an option for treating adults who stammer. As such we advocate that every specialist clinician should be able to offer this to their clients. However, not all clinicians have enough adult clients on their caseload to be able to do this. In these instances we recommend that clinicians work collaboratively with others in neighbouring districts or regions. In this way they can combine resources and 'manpower', while clients have the opportunity to meet together and may go on to set up self-help meetings in a central location after therapy has ended.

Selection. Groups of clients need to be selected to attend for group therapy. Initially, there should be some selection criteria which function to reduce possible problems. Examples of criteria to consider are as follows:

- hearing problems
- visual difficulties
- cognitive and learning difficulties
- mental illness
- difficulties with social interaction
- poor concentration and limited attention span
- reading and writing problems
- other difficulties which make understanding language difficult.

Note that we are not suggesting that adults who stammer and who have additional problems are not suitable candidates for group therapy. On the contrary, some groups we have run in the past have included clients with a range of the issues listed above. We are merely pointing out that these issues need careful consideration in the context of a group therapy programme.

In relation to the presentation of stammering, obviously there will be shared areas of difficulty. However, some specialist centres in England offer groups for adults with primarily overt issues and other sessions for clients with primarily covert-based difficulties. Again, not having enough of each type may prevent some clinicians from doing this. Nevertheless, in the past we have been able to run groups incorporating individuals with vastly different types of stammering. In these instances, sometimes the clients with more covert features may feel the need to 'explain' why they do not overtly stammer to the other group members. If this is done early on in the group the feelings of difference can be managed and the group will gel appropriately.

Organisation. There are various ways in which groups can run:

- Some groups run with a fixed start and end point with all clients progressing through the same activities and tasks together. These types of group are useful for teaching a specific skill such as block modification or assertiveness.
- Other types of group can be more flexible, with individuals joining and/or leaving the group at any point. People progress through the process of the group at their own pace and acquire a diverse range of skills and knowledge on the way. One of the benefits of running a group where clients are at different stages is being able to use the group wisdom. In this context a 'sage' is someone who has successfully managed a particular process and can be asked to contribute his ideas to help another group member. For example, Mick, who uses voluntary stammering in several contexts, will be asked to introduce and explain how to use it to a group member who is new to the idea. This validates the progress Mick has made as

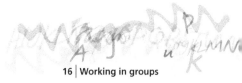

well as adding to the understanding of the newer member by providing a real-life example. It also enables the clients to come to view themselves as the experts rather than the clinicians.

- In some groups the content of the sessions is determined by the members who attend. This can be managed by having the group share ideas or options at predetermined intervals, for example, every 12 weeks. The group then prioritises the topics generated, and plans for the time period are developed using these ideas. A written timetable will then be provided for the group so the clients see what has been agreed and when the topics will take place, and consider what they need to do in preparation.

- In other groups the content is predetermined, usually by the leader or clinician. This type of group would be useful for developing skills such as identification.

Clients need to be at the same stage. We do not mean necessarily that all group members will be at the same point in the process of therapy while attending group sessions; that will depend on the type of group that is in place. We *do* mean that clients need to be in an action phase of change (see Prochaska & DiClemente's stages of change in Chapter 1) and to start at a similar point when they enter the group. Each client joining our group programme is likely to have completed work on variation and identification. In this way he will have a shared knowledge and understanding of his stammer and a shared vocabulary with the other group members.

Common problems

Attendance and late arrival. Attendance can be erratic. It is essential for the group to gel and develop as a supportive unit for there to be a coherent and consistent group of regulars who attend on time. For this reason we are very strict about attendance. We specify at the outset of joining the group, usually when agreeing ground rules, that we expect individuals to prioritise the group for several months and we set a 'three strikes and out' rule (that is, if a client misses three meetings without letting the group know, he loses his place in the group). We also explain how people can inform other group members or us if they are not coming, otherwise the group will wait for them. (Acceptable reasons for not attending include nuclear holocaust, tsunami, death or other serious illness! However, we will always try to contact clients who have missed sessions to find out if there are any issues we can help with.)

Venue. It is important to meet at an appropriate location, but finding somewhere suitable can be difficult. The venue needs to be a central point readily accessible by transport networks. We recommend a setting that strikes a balance between the formal and the informal. A pub is too informal and a hospital or community clinic can be too formal. It is useful to be able to provide refreshments as this will help to develop a more relaxed, informal atmosphere. Security can be an issue when meeting in the evening, so it is important to ensure that any security staff are aware of the start and finish time of the session.

Integrating new members. Meeting as a group for the first time or joining an established group can be a daunting experience for all of us. For an adult who stammers the anxiety can be heightened, knowing that he will have to speak in front of these new people. It is helpful to explain to a client before he joins that, as his clinician, you can introduce him to the group if he wishes, saying his name and any other details he might agree to share at that stage. This reduces the pressure and we often find it enables the person to say a bit more at the time than he initially thought he would be able to.

Where we have two or more clients wanting to join a group at the same time, rather than take them through identification in individual therapy, we will run a mini group (over the course of a day) on identification. This will then enable them to join the existing therapy group at the same time and feel more comfortable because they are already familiar with at least one other person in the group.

In the first and early sessions clinicians should listen keenly for any vocabulary or terminology that might be unfamiliar to new members. In these instances existing group members can be invited to explain these terms, thus confirming their roles as experts in the group.

It is also important not to have 'major' activities planned for the first session or two of a new member's attendance, for example, doing a survey. This can be too threatening for individuals trying to get to grips with participating in a group and the demands on their communication.

Difficult clients. Some clients can be difficult to integrate into groups. Here are some examples of roles to look out for:

'I'm not like any of you.'

'Just tell me what to do and I will do it.'

'My family/work colleagues don't understand me.'

'Yes, but ...'

'I need to tell you all about this. And it's going to take a long time.'

'I think stammering is very amusing and I often laugh at others who stammer.'

Individuals with overt and covert stammering in the same group. As we have stated earlier in this chapter, we run groups in which clients with primarily overt stammering sit alongside those with covert-based difficulties. We would reiterate here the need in such situations for clients with more covert features to introduce their type of stammering to the group from the outset. It can easily be carried out in the context of a 'Stammer like me manual' or other activity in which a client describes in detail his particular stammer and the impact it has on his life.

Gender imbalance. As we know, there are more males who stammer than females. This usually results in a greater number of men in groups. It is always valuable to have women in the group as the dynamic changes and different perspectives emerge. However, sometimes there might only be one woman in a group of six or seven men and that can be difficult. If there are two or three women, the issues are more manageable. If there is only one woman, it is appropriate to let her make her own decision about attending the group.

Time keeping. Giving every group member equal amounts of time to talk in a group can be problematic. It is essential to have a clock visible and for responsibility for time keeping to be shared among group members.

Group bravery. Being in a group can help a client to feel brave, to take risks that he would not normally have considered and do things he would not normally do on his own. However, once the client leaves the group, then, without an appropriate level of support, he may lose his confidence to continue the change process.

Significant other people and the group. As we have stated earlier, the change in the individual can cause some issues in his relationships. This may have implications for roles, especially within a couple (see Chapter 15 'Maintenance: a continuing process of change'). Consequently, clinicians need to involve significant others as early as possible in the process and discuss with them the implications of therapy and the process of change.

Leaving the group. The group can become a very comfortable and secure place. Sometimes a client might need to be given a push to leave. The development of the toolbox can be useful in this regard. The process of drawing it together, having a draft commented on, setting a date for presentation and then the more formal 'ceremony' of presenting can lead the client towards a closure point. Occasionally a client will avoid closure by attending more erratically as the leaving date approaches. In these instances it is important to continue to be firm about attendance and stress the importance of the group hearing his toolbox.

Ideas for working in a group

These are some of the ideas and activities we have found useful in the groups we run.

Ground rules. It is essential for the group to set ground rules at the outset and/or when new members join. Typically, these can include rules about:

- listening to others
- turn taking, not interrupting
- supporting others
- managing stammering (how both difficult overt episodes and covert issues such as avoidance might be managed in the group)
- being open and honest
- maintaining confidentiality
- attendance (and how to let members know if a person is unable to attend)
- other: for example, mobile phones, refreshments.

Cue cards. A client will choose two or three cards that represent aspects of communication he is working on in the group situation. Examples might include:

- maintaining good eye contact
- upright posture
- using an appropriate speech rate
- using voluntary stammering
- moving forward in an utterance (that is, not going back over dysfluent words or having a run into a word)
- using easy onset
- using light contacts.

Each card has a symbol or written word representing the target and a positive affirmation of the target on the reverse side.

A client distributes his chosen cards to other group members at the start of the evening, thereby asking them to monitor that particular aspect of his communication. These are used as an alternative to interrupting a speaker in the middle of what he is saying, to remind him of a target or technique he should be using. During his verbal contribution group members

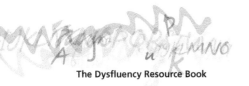

will hold up the card when they think the client is falling short of achieving his desired target. Alternatively, they can flip the card over, signifying to the individual that he is achieving his aim and doing well.

Fines. Losing money is a great motivator! In our group clients are encouraged to set themselves a target of a number of voluntary stammers to achieve in a group therapy session. If the target is not met the person will pay double the target sum in pence. Occasionally, the regime is altered to encourage the whole group to support each other in achieving a target. For example, the whole group may be required to pay if any one member of the group does not achieve his target. (The fines are collected and sent to the British Stammering Association, usually with a letter of explanation written by a group member!) A further variation on this theme stipulates that anyone failing to meet his target is required to buy a group member who has been successful in reaching their target their favourite chocolate bar.

Introductory exercise. At the beginning of a group session clients will take it in turns to lead an introductory task. This contributes to the feeling that they can facilitate the group and it enables each client to practise presenting in front of a group. This always includes a person saying his name, listing the features of communication he plans to work on during the session and completing a short task. Examples of short tasks for this introduction to the evening are for each group member (clients and clinician) to talk about one of the following topics:

- Three people you would invite to dinner

- Your favourite place to live

- A historical figure you would like to have been

- A period in history you would like to have lived through

- A musical instrument you would like to play

- Three everyday items you would take to a desert island

- Where your first name comes from

- Which animal, bird or fish you would choose to be, and why

- A funny childhood memory.

Resources. It is important to have a good supply of information leaflets, handouts on techniques, monitoring sheets and so on ready to hand. In addition, we have a range of self-help books that we loan out, and information on the British Stammering Association.

For those starting to write up their toolbox (see Chapter 15 'Maintenance: a continuing process of change') we hold a file of copies of toolboxes presented previously so that clients can get some ideas for their own. (We always ask a client who presents his toolbox for permission to keep a copy of it in this file. We have never had anyone refuse and often a client will come prepared with a copy for the file.)

Work on transitions. It is important to provide some support for clients who leave the group. The move from good support to no support will not help an individual maintain the change he has made. However, providing some level of support, albeit not to the same degree as a therapy group, can help facilitate this change. If there is a self-help group operating in the area it is useful to set up joint meetings or get-togethers from time to time. In this way clients get to know other group members, which makes the transition from therapy group to self-help group easier. Alternatively, representatives from self-help groups can be invited along to a therapy group to introduce themselves and describe their meetings, programme, structure, venue and so on.

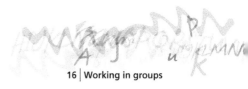

Phone tree. Group members are formally asked to exchange phone/mobile numbers. This simple activity has several benefits in that it:

• reduces isolation

• encourages work on targeted areas between members

• moves work on targets to *outside* the group setting

• facilitates group support

• develops a social network among group members.

Useful sessions

Throughout the chapters of this book we have indicated activities that are suitable for group sessions (shown by 🎇). We would like to underline this further by listing tasks we particularly recommend.

Survey: Chapter 7

Dealing with difficult listeners: Chapter 7

Speaking circles: Chapter 7

Situation role play: one particularly useful situation to role play is an interview. Where group members have debated the pros and cons of mentioning their stammering when involved in a recruitment process we have on occasions invited a personnel officer to attend the group and discuss his perspective.

Presentations by clients telling their own life story or narrative.

In addition, we always include *significant other evenings* in any planned period of group therapy. This is a session where each group member is required to bring another person to the group. This person is important to them in some way and may be a close relative, partner, friend or work colleague. Clients choose to bring certain people for a variety of reasons. It might be someone who they particularly wish to know about the difficulties of stammering or someone close to them who would be a good support in working on their speech. A couple of weeks before the session we ask group members to decide on the format and content of the evening. This enables them to work on the specific issues they have, be it creating support or dispelling myths about stammering. We also ask them to consider the practicalities of splitting the group into smaller units, for example, putting the 'significant others' together in a group, separating the significant other from the person who brought them, and so on. In considering these issues they often come to realise that people without communication problems also may find meeting new people and talking in group settings difficult.

There are a number of ideas that have emerged over time which we would recommend to readers who have not run these types of session before:

• Group members (individually or in pairs) explain speech techniques to small groups of visitors.

• Group members complete a group iceberg on stammering in front of the significant others.

• Small groups of clients sit in different rooms and the significant others can move about and 'visit' the rooms and find out about various topics, for example, information about stammering, describing the features of stammering (overt and covert issues), society's view of stammering.

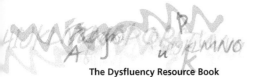

• Have a discussion about the advantages and disadvantages of stammering.

We would always allow some time within this type of session for the clients to outline to the group of visitors how best to help in situations where stammering occurs.

Details of a session plan for such an evening are given below.

'Significant others' attending a group therapy session ⚙

Each group member introduces the person he has brought to the group and says why he chose to invite them. Clinicians explain the aims of the group and what has been carried out to date.

Two small groups are formed, with group members joining a different group from their significant other or partner. Each adult who stammers describes his stammer and makes a statement on 'What I have learned so far' or 'How I have changed'.

Each group is given a statement on stammering to discuss. One group member makes notes during the small-group discussion and feeds back to the large group at the end of the discussion.

The following are examples of discussion topics to be used (adapted from Sheehan 1958, 1975).

1 Stammering is a false role disorder. You will remain a person who has a stammer as long as you continue to pretend not to be one.

2 Your stammering is something you do, not something that happens to you. It is your behaviour, not a condition.

3 What you call your stammering consists mostly of the tricks and strategies you use to cover it up. It is far better to stammer openly and honestly than it is to use a trick, even if it is temporarily successful.

4 In accepting yourself as a person who has a stammer, you choose the route to becoming a more honest, relaxed speaker. The more you run away from your stammering, the more you will stammer. The more you are open and courageous, the more you will develop good communication.

5 Your fear of stammering is based largely on your shame and hatred of it. The fear is also based on playing the phony role in which you pretend your stuttering doesn't exist. You can do something about this fear if you have the courage. You can be open about your stammering above the surface. You can learn to go ahead and speak anyway, going forward in the face of fear.

6 Perfect fluency is not obtainable and is a self-defeating goal.

7 You may be astonished that fluency is anything to which you would have to adjust. Yet it is a central problem in the consolidation of improvement.

At the end of the session there is an opportunity for people to ask the therapy group members questions.

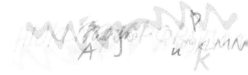

References

Alm PA (2004) 'Stuttering and the basal ganglia circuits', *Journal of Communication Disorders,* 37, pp325–69.

Beck AT, Emery G & Greenberg RL (1985) *Anxiety Disorders and Phobias: A Cognitive Perspective,* Basic Books, New York.

Beck AT (1993) *Cognitive Therapy and the Emotional Disorders,* Penguin, New York.

Bennett-Levy J, Westbrook D, Fennell M, Cooper M, Rouf K & Hackman A (2004) 'Behavioural experiments: historical and conceptual underpinnings', Bennett-Levy J, Butler G, Fennell M, Hackman A, Mueller M & Westbrook D (eds), *Oxford Guide to Behavioural Experiments in Cognitive Therapy,* Oxford University Press, Oxford.

Blenkiron P (2007) 'Change view', *CBT Today,* 36 (3), p2.

Bloodstein O (1969, 1975) *A Handbook on Stuttering,* 1st & 2nd edns, National Easter Seal Society for Crippled Children and Adults, Chicago, IL.

Bloodstein O (1995) *A Handbook on Stuttering,* 5th edn, Chapman & Hall, London.

Boone DR, McFarlane SC & Von Berg SL (2005) *The Voice and Voice Therapy,* 7th edn, Pearson, Boston, MA.

Bonnard M (1996) Personal communication, St James University Hospital, Leeds.

Borkovec TD & Costello E (1993) 'Efficacy of applied relaxation and cognitive behavioural therapy in the treatment of generalised anxiety disorder', *Journal of Consulting & Clinical Psychology,* 61, pp611–19.

Bothe AK (2004) 'Evidence-based practice in stuttering treatment: an introduction', Bothe AK (ed), *Evidence-Based Treatment of Stuttering: Empirical Bases and Clinical Applications,* Lawrence Erlbaum Associates, Mahwah, NJ.

Bourne EJ (2005) *The Anxiety and Phobia Workbook,* 4th edn, New Harbinger Workbooks, Oakland, CA.

Brutten EJ & Shoemaker DJ (1967) *The Modification of Stuttering*, Prentice Hall, Englewood Cliffs, NJ.

Button E (1985) *Personal Construct Theory & Mental Health,* Croom Helm, London.

Cheasman C (2007) 'Revealing and healing: a mindfulness approach to stammering', *Speaking Out,* Spring, pp9–10.

Cooper EB (1979) 'Intervention procedures for the young stutterer', Gregory HH (ed), *Controversies about Stuttering Therapy,* University Park Press, Baltimore, MD.

Corcoran J & Stewart M (1998) 'Stories of stuttering: a qualitative analysis of interview narratives', *Journal of Fluency Disorders,* 23, pp247–64.

Craig AR (1986) 'The prevention and prediction of relapse following behavior therapy for stuttering', unpublished doctoral thesis, University of New South Wales, Sydney.

Dalton P (1994) *Counselling People with Communication Problems,* Sage, London.

Dalton P & Dunnett G (1989) *A Psychology for Living,* Dunton Publishing, London.

de Shazer S (1985) *Keys to Solution in Brief Therapy,* Norton, New York.

de Shazer S (1988) *Clues: Investigating Solutions in Brief Therapy,* Norton, New York.

DiClemente CC (1991) 'Motivational interviewing and the stages of change', Miller WR & Rollnick S (eds), *Motivational Interviewing,* Guilford Press, New York.

Douglas E & Quarrington B (1952) 'The differentiation of interiorized and exteriorized secondary stuttering', *Journal of Speech & Hearing Disorders,* 17, pp377–85.

Eisenson J (1975) 'Stuttering as perseverative behaviour', Eisenson J (ed), *Stuttering: A Second Symposium,* Harper & Row, New York.

Evesham M & Fransella F (1985) 'Stuttering relapse: the effect of a combined speech and psychological reconstruction programme', *International Journal of Language & Communication Disorders,* 20 (3) pp237–48.

Finn P (2003) 'Evidence-based treatment of stuttering. II Clinical significance of behavioral stuttering treatments', *Journal of Fluency Disorders,* 28 (3), pp209–18.

Fransella F (1972) *Personal Change and Reconstruction: Research on a Treatment of Stuttering,* Academic Press, London.

Fransella F & Dalton P (1990) *Personal Construct Counselling in Action,* Sage, London.

Fraser M (2007) *Self-therapy for the Stutterer,* 10th edn, Stuttering Foundation of America, Publication No.12, Memphis, TN.

Glickstein L (1989) *Be Heard Now,* Broadway Books, New York.

Greer R (1991) 'Hypnosis and stammering', *Speaking Out,* Winter, p6.

Gregory HH (1979) 'Controversial issues: statement and review of the literature', Gregory HH (ed), *Controversies about Stuttering Therapy,* University Park Press, Baltimore, MD.

Hayhow R & Levy C (1989) *Working with Stuttering,* Winslow Press, Bicester, Oxon.

Hargie O (2006) *The Handbook of Communication Skills,* 3rd edn, Routledge, East Sussex.

Harrison J (2000) *Redefining Stuttering: What the Struggle to Speak is Really About,* 12th edn, National Stuttering Association, Anaheim Hills, CA.

Jackson S (1989) 'Self-characterisation: dimensions of meaning', Fransella F & Thomas L (eds), *Experimenting with Personal Construct Psychology,* Routledge & Kegan Paul, London & New York.

Kabat-Zinn J (1994) *Wherever You Go, There You Are: Mindfulness Meditation in Everyday Life,* Hyperion, New York.

Kelly GA (1991) *The Psychology of Personal Constructs,* 2nd edn, Routledge, London.

Kuhr A (1991) 'Should all adults be treated?', *Human Communication,* November, pp17–19.

Lambert MJ & Barley DE (2001) 'Research summary on the therapeutic relationship and psychotherapy outcome', *Psychotherapy,* 38 (4), pp357–61.

Levy L (1987) 'Interiorised stuttering: a group therapy approach', Levy C (ed), *Stuttering Therapy: Practical Approaches*, Croom Helm, London.

Logan J & Sheasby S (2007) 'Using therapeutic writing to support a client's new story', *Signal,* 27, pp2–3.

Luper HL & Mulder RL (1964) *Stuttering: Therapy for Children,* Prentice Hall, Englewood Cliffs, NJ.

Manning WH (2000) *Clinical Decision Making in Fluency Disorders,* 2nd edn, Singular, Vancouver.

Mathieson L (2001) *Greene and Mathieson's The Voice and its Disorders,* 6th edn, Wiley, New Jersey.

Martin S & Lockhart M (2000) *Working with Voice Disorders,* Winslow, Bicester, Oxon.

Norcross JC & Prochaska CC (1986) 'Psychologist heal thyself. 1 The psychological distress and self change of psychologists, counselors and lay persons', *Psychotherapy*, 23, pp102–14.

O'Hanlon W & Weiner-Davis M (1989) *In Search of Solutions,* WW Norton, New York.

Payne RA (1995) *Relaxation Techniques,* Churchill Livingstone, London.

Prochaska JO & DiClemente CC (1986) 'Towards a comprehensive model of change', Miller WE & Heather N (eds), *Handbook of Eclectic Therapy,* Plenum Press, New York.

Prochaska JO & DiClemente CC (1992) 'Stages of change in the modification of problem behaviours', Herson M, Eisler RM & Miller PM (eds), *Progress in Behaviour Modification,* 28, Sycamore, IL.

Royal College of Speech & Language Therapists (2006) *Communicating Quality 3: RCSLT's Guidance on Best Practice in Service Organisation and Provision,* London.

Ryan B & Van Kirk B (1971) *Monterey Fluency Program,* Monterey Learning Systems, Palo Alto, CA.

Segal ZV, Williams JMG & Teasdale JD (2002) *Mindfulness-Based Cognitive Therapy for Depression: A New Approach to Preventing Relapse,* Guilford Press, New York.

Sheehan JG (1958) 'Conflict theory and avoidance reduction therapy', Eisenson J & Bloodstein O (eds), *Stuttering: A Symposium,* Harper, New York.

Sheehan JG (1975) 'Conflict theory and avoidance reduction therapy', Eisenson J (ed), *Stuttering: A Second Symposium,* Harper & Row, New York.

Sheehan JG (1979) 'Stuttering and recovery', Gregory HH (ed), *Controversies about Stuttering Therapy,* University Park Press, Baltimore, MD.

Sheehan JG (1983) Excerpts from the writings of Joseph G Sheehan, memorial service, 26 November 1983, British Stammering Association, London.

Sheehan VM (1980) 'Approach-avoidance and anxiety reduction', Shames GH & Rubin HR (eds), *Stuttering Then and Now,* Charles E Merrill Publishing Company, Columbus, OH.

Snaith RP (1974) 'A method of psychotherapy based on relaxation techniques', *British Journal of Psychiatry,* 124, pp473–8.

Snaith RP (1981) *Clinical Neurosis,* Oxford University Press, Oxford.

Stewart T (1996) 'Good maintainers and poor maintainers: a personal construct approach to an old problem', *Journal of Fluency Disorders,* 21, pp 22–48.

Stewart T (2005) 'The artist's eye', keynote presentation at the Oxford Dysfluency Conference, Oxford.

Stewart T & Birdsall M (2001) 'A review of the contribution of personal construct psychology to stammering therapy', *Journal of Constructivist Psychology,* 14 (3), pp 215–25.

Stewart T & Brosh H (1997) 'The use of drawing in the management of adults who stammer', *Journal of Fluency Disorders,* 22 (1), pp35–50.

Stewart T & Richardson G (2004) 'A qualitative study of therapeutic effect from a user's perspective', *Journal of Fluency Disorders,* 29, pp95–108.

Stewart T & Turnbull J (2007) *Working with Dysfluent Children,* Speechmark, Bicester, Oxon.

Stuttering Foundation of America (1995) *To the Stutterer,* Publication No. 9, Memphis, TN.

Sunderland M & Engleheart P (1993) *Draw on Your Emotions,* Winslow Press, Bicester, Oxon.

Thorne B (1990) 'Person-centred therapy', Dryden W (ed), *Individual Therapy: A Handbook,* Open University Press, Milton Keynes.

Turnbull J (2000) 'The Transtheoretical Model of Change: examples from stammering', *Counselling Psychology Quarterly,* 13 (1), pp13–21.

Van Riper C (1973) *The Treatment of Stuttering,* Prentice Hall, Englewood Cliffs, NJ.

Van Riper C (1982) *The Nature of Stuttering,* Prentice Hall, Englewood Cliffs, NJ.

Van Riper C (1986) 'Modification of behaviour. Part two', Shames GH & Rubin HR (eds), *Stuttering Then and Now,* Charles E Merrill Publishing Company, Columbus, OH.

Van Riper C (1990) 'Final thoughts about stuttering', *Journal of Fluency Disorders,* 15, pp317–18.

Ward D (2006) *Stuttering and Cluttering: Frameworks for Understanding and Treatment,* Taylor & Francis/Psychology Press, Hove, Sussex.

Webster RL (1974) 'A behavioral analysis of stuttering: treatment and theory', Calhoun KS, Adams HE & Mitchell KM (eds), *Innovative Treatment Methods in Psychopathology,* Wiley, New York.

Webster WG & Poulos MG (1989) *Facilitating Fluency: Transfer Strategies for Adult Stuttering Treatment Programs,* Communication Skill Builders, Tucson, AZ.

Wells A (1995) 'Meta-cognition and worry: a cognitive model of generalised anxiety disorder', *Behavioural and Cognitive Psychotherapy,* 23, pp301–20.

Williams DE (1979) 'A perspective on approaches to stuttering therapy', Gregory HH (ed), *Controversies about Stuttering Therapy,* University Park Press, Baltimore, MD.

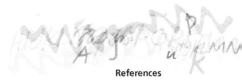

Williams R (1995) 'Personal construct theory in use with people who stutter', Fawcus M (ed), *Stuttering from Theory to Practice,* Whurr Publishers, London.

Zigmond AS & Snaith RP (1983) 'Hospital anxiety and depression scale', *Acta Psychiatrica Scandinavia,* 67, pp361–70.

Websites

British Stammering Association, www.stammering.org

Living Life to the Full, www.livinglifetothefull.com

Stuttering Foundation of America, www.stutteringhelp.org

T - #0006 - 160425 - C0 - 297/210/13 - WB - 9780863887925 - Gloss Lamination